You...

C000256491

Knee Replacement

Jane Smith BSc *(Hons)*

Medical Editor and Writer, Bristol

&

Ian D. Learmonth FRCS, FRCS *(Ed)*, FCS *(SA) Orth*

Professor and Head of the Department of Orthopaedic Surgery,
University of Bristol

ILLUSTRATIONS BY ALEXANDER JAMES

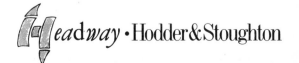

Headway · Hodder & Stoughton

Other titles published in this series

Breast Lumps
Hernias
Hysterectomy & alternative operations
Varicose Veins
Male and Female Sterilisation
Cataracts
Skin Cancers
Prostate Problems
Hip Replacement

A catalogue record for this title is available from the British Library.

ISBN 0 340 679093

First published 1997
Impression number   10 9 8 7 6 5 4 3 2 1
Year   1999 1998 1997

Typeset by Wearset, Boldon, Tyne and Wear
Printed in Great Britain for Hodder & Stoughton Educational, a division of Hodder Headline Plc, 338 Euston Road, London NW1 3BH by Cox & Wyman Ltd, Reading, Berks.

Contents

General preface to the series

Two people having the same operation can have quite different experiences, but one feeling that is common to many is that things might have been easier if they had had a better idea of what to expect. Some people are reluctant to ask questions, and many forget what they are told, sometimes because they are anxious, and sometimes because they do not really understand the explanations they are given.

In most medical centres in Britain today, the emphasis is more on patient involvement than at any time in the past. It is now generally accepted that it is important for people to understand what their treatment entails, both in terms of reducing their stress and thus aiding their recovery, and of making their care more straightforward for the medical staff involved.

The books in this series have been written with the aim of giving people comprehensive information about each of the medical conditions covered, about the treatment they are likely to be offered, and about what may happen during their post-operative recovery period. Armed with this knowledge, you should have the confidence to question, and to take part in the decisions made.

Going in to hospital for the first time can be a daunting experience, and therefore the books describe the procedures involved, and identify and explain the roles of the hospital staff with whom you are likely to come into contact.

Anaesthesia is explained in general terms, and the options

available for a particular operation are described in each book.

There may be complications following any operation – usually minor but none the less worrying for the person involved – and the common ones are described and explained. Now that less time is spent in hospital following most non-emergency operations, knowing what to expect in the days following surgery, and what to do if a complication does arise, is more important than ever before.

Where relevant, the books include a section of exercises and advice to help you to get back to normal and to deal with the everyday activities which can be difficult or painful in the first few days after an operation.

Doctors and nurses, like members of any profession, use a jargon, and they often forget that many of the terms that are familiar to them are not part of everyday language for most of us. Care has been taken to make the books easily understandable by everyone, and each book has a list of simple explanations of the medical terms you may come across.

Most doctors and nurses are more than willing to explain and to discuss problems with patients, but they often assume that if you do not ask questions, you either do not want to know or you know already. Questions and answers are given in every book to help you to draw up your own list to take with you when you see your family doctor or consultant.

Each book also has a section of case histories of people who have experienced the particular operation themselves. These are included to give you an idea of the problems which can arise, problems which may sometimes seem relatively trivial to others but which can be distressing to those directly concerned.

Although the majority of people are satisfied with the medical care they receive, things can go wrong. If you do feel you need to make a complaint about something that happened, or did not happen, during your treatment, each book has a section which deals in detail with how to go about this.

It was the intention in writing these books to help to take some of the worry out of having an operation. It is not knowing what to expect, and the feeling of being involved in some process over which we have no control, and which we do not fully understand, that makes us anxious. The books in the series *Your Operation* should help to remove some of that anxiety and make you feel less like a car being serviced, and more like part of the team of people who are working together to cure your medical problem and put you back on the road to health.

You may not know *all* there is to know about a particular condition when you have read the book related to it, but you will know more than enough to prepare yourself for your operation. You may decide you do not want to go ahead with surgery. Although this is not the authors' intention, they will be happy that you have been given enough information to feel confident to make your own decision, and to take an active part in your own care. After all, it is *your* operation.

Jane Smith
Bristol, 1997

Preface

Most people undergoing total knee replacement are in the older age group, but the operation is also sometimes suitable for younger people and can transform the life of someone who has suffered pain and disability, possibly for many years. However, it is major surgery and it does require serious commitment to the post-operative exercises necessary to regain strength and mobility in the knee joint. Therefore it is important that anyone contemplating knee replacement has a clear understanding of what it involves and of the part they themselves must play in their rehabilitation during the months following surgery.

It is vital that you follow the specific advice and instructions given to you by your doctor to enable you to make the fullest possible recovery after your operation and to regain maximum mobility in your knee. By describing all that is involved in knee replacement surgery, this book helps explain the reasons for the advice you will be given. Complications can occur after any type of surgery and explanations are given of the most common ones to help both patients and their carers recognise the signs for which medical attention should be sought.

Despite our use of the word 'you' when referring to 'the patient', the book has also been written for the friends, relatives and other carers whose need for information is sometimes overlooked.

Jane Smith
Ian D. Learmonth
Bristol, 1997

Acknowledgements

We are grateful to all the people who gave so generously of their time and knowledge to help in the writing of this book. Particular thanks are due to Ward Sister Thelma Richards, to Lesley Roper (Superintendent Physiotherapist), to Meg Birch (Occupational Therapy Services Manager), and to Maureen Lee (Research Assistant, University of Bristol), all at the Avon Orthopaedic Centre, Southmead Hospital, Bristol.

Special thanks go to the men and women who related their own experiences for the section of case histories.

CHAPTER 1

Introduction

There has been considerable advance both in surgical techniques and in the instrumentation used for total knee replacement since the operation first began to be practised about 30 years ago. However, it is only fairly recently that the long-term results of total knee replacement have become known: good results, with the replaced knee still functioning satisfactorily 15 years after the operation, are achieved in some 90 per cent of cases. There has been an increase in the number of operations performed, and approximately 30 000 in the UK and over 250 000 in the USA are now carried out each year. Total knee replacement is already more common than hip replacement in the USA, and a similar trend is also apparent in the UK.

Most people undergoing total knee replacement tend to be in the older age group; those having surgery because of damage to the knee joint due to osteoarthritis are mainly in their late sixties or older. However, many people with joint destruction due to rheumatoid arthritis have a knee joint replaced in their forties or fifties.

It is possible for someone suffering from another illness to undergo knee replacement surgery provided the approval of the appropriate specialist is obtained. Therefore, for example, anyone with heart disease will be referred to a heart specialist for examination before knee surgery is agreed to.

Knee replacement operations are primarily carried out to relieve pain and to restore movement and stability to the knee joint, and there are many different causes of painful arthritis at this site. Sometimes both knees need to be replaced, and whereas this may involve two separate operations, six weeks to three months apart, bilateral surgery (when both joints are replaced at the same time) is not uncommon (see p.14).

Although surgery can dramatically improve the pain and restricted mobility caused by damage, disease or degeneration of the knee joint, it is not appropriate in all cases. Therefore, before a decision can be made to go ahead with an operation, it is important that a full assessment is made to determine the cause of the problem and to make sure there is nothing in the individual's medical or social history which could affect the operation itself, the use of anaesthesia or the rehabilitation process afterwards. It is very important that anyone contemplating total knee replacement understands the part they themselves must play in their rehabilitation to ensure that adequate muscle power and as full a range of movement as possible are regained in the knee joint. A physiotherapist will demonstrate the various exercises and assist with the rehabilitation programme, advising on any special physiotherapy that may be required. However, it is the responsibility of the individual to do the exercises regularly. Without them, an operation may cure the pain but poor muscle control, loss of movement and an inability to straighten the knee fully may result in permanent disability. Good motivation and commitment to post-operative rehabilitation are therefore essential.

Total knee replacement is a major operation and should only be considered when other treatments have proved, or seem likely to prove, ineffective. Although a doctor or consultant can explain the probable outcome of surgery in a particular case, the individual concerned must make the final decision. To do so, it is necessary not only to understand what is involved in the operation and the possible complications which could occur, but also to have realistic expectations about its outcome. It is hoped that this book will provide enough information to help people make the right decision for themselves, and that it will be a useful source of reference to members of their families and anyone else involved in their post-operative care.

MEDICAL TERMS

Explanations of some of the medical terms you may come across in any discussion of knee replacement surgery are given below. Others are explained in Appendix III on page 116.

Arthropathy is any disease which affects a joint. **Arthroplasty** is an operation to alleviate pain and restore the function of a joint by cutting out the damaged bone and, in most cases, replacing it with an artificial component, known as a **prosthesis**. There are different types of knee arthroplasty but this book concentrates on **total knee replacement** which involves the complete replacement of the upper end of the calf bone and of the lower end of the thigh bone with which it articulates. It may or may not also include replacement of the knee cap.

Hemi-arthroplasty involves basically the same operation, but only one half of the joint is replaced, usually the inner (**medial**) part of the ends of the calf and thigh bones. Knee hemi-arthroplasty is undertaken in selected cases and can be a useful operation for younger people because it is relatively straightforward to revise it to a total knee replacement at a later date if necessary. Alternatively, it offers an option of more limited surgery for older people in whom only one side of the knee is involved.

Other types of surgery for arthritis of the knee include **osteotomy**, which involves cutting through either the calf bone or the thigh bone to alter the alignment and thus the direction of force exerted across the joint on walking. The knee may also be 'cleaned out' to remove fragments of cartilage and other debris, although the benefits of this process of **debridement** are usually short lived.

Arthrodesis is the surgical fusion of bones to produce a completely rigid, inflexible joint. It may be considered as a way of providing stability and abolishing pain for a young person with no problems in any other joints, although it does so at the expense of mobility. It is also sometimes used as a salvage procedure following removal of the implant after failure of total knee replacement.

THE KNEE JOINT

To understand what happens when the knee joint becomes diseased or damaged, it is helpful to know something of its anatomy and function.

The calf – the lower part of the leg between the knee and the ankle – consists of two bones: an inner, thicker, strong bone called the **tibia**, and an outer, thinner **fibula**. Above the knee there is a single thigh bone, called the **femur**. The knee joint is a type of **hinge joint** (although not a true one) and is formed where the flattened upper end of the tibia articulates with two rounded **condyles** at the lower end of the femur. The knee cap, known as the **patella**, is a small bone which lies in front of the knee and mechanically improves the performance of the muscles on the front of the thigh which straighten the knee.

The articulating surfaces of the tibia and femur are covered by **articular cartilage**, a highly specialised load-bearing tissue with a very low coefficient of friction. The semi-lunar **menisci** ('cartilages'; singular: **meniscus**) interposed between the articular surfaces of the femur and tibia increase the contact area between

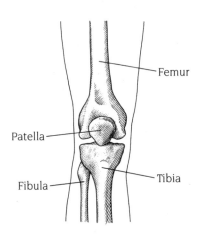

The bones of the knee.

4

the two bones, thus decreasing the load on the joint surface.

Attached to the rim of the cartilage is a **capsule** of strong, fibrous tissue. Parts of the capsule tissue are thickened to form **ligaments** which support the bones of the joint and prevent them dislocating during normal movement. The knee joint also has a rich supply of blood vessels, lymph vessels and nerves, and is surrounded by muscles which control its movement (see below) and contribute to stability. Because the bones at the joint are relatively unconstrained, strong ligaments and muscles are essential to maintain stability in the knee.

The knee joint is a **synovial joint**. The inner surface of the capsule is lined with **synovium**, a membrane of specialised tissue which secretes an oily **synovial fluid** to lubricate the joint and allow for smooth movement of its parts.

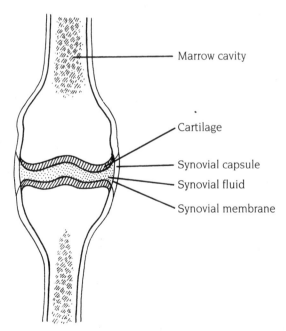

Marrow cavity

Cartilage

Synovial capsule

Synovial fluid

Synovial membrane

A typical synovial joint.

Movement of the knee joint

When stimulated by a nervous impulse, muscle cells contract, making the muscle shorter. As the muscle shortens, it pulls on the bones and produces movement. The muscles across joints such as the knee act as levers: by contracting only a few centimetres they can produce movement in the limb of tens of centimetres.

As muscles cannot lengthen beyond their relaxed, resting length, they are normally present in pairs: contraction of one muscle of the pair produces movement in one direction, whereas contraction of the other produces movement in the opposite direction. Around the knee joint, these **antagonistic pairs** of muscles act to extend and flex the leg, i.e. to straighten and bend it. Flexion is controlled by the **hamstring muscles** which run down behind the knee and which include the **biceps femoris**, the **semitendinosus** and the **semimembranosus** muscles. Extension is controlled by the **quadriceps femoris muscle** at the front of the knee. The tibia is also able to rotate, both internally and externally, in relation to the femur.

Some or all of these movements may be lost following long-term joint disease, and the soft tissues and muscles around the joint will then shorten, leading to **contracture**. The most common problem following disease of the knee joint is **flexion contracture**: the joint can bend but cannot be fully straightened.

CAUSES OF PROBLEMS WITH THE KNEE JOINT

There are several problems and diseases which can affect the knee joint (as well as other joints in the body), causing damage to the bones and other tissues and eventually pain and reduced mobility. The more severe the pain and disability suffered before surgery, the more dramatic its effects are likely to be. Osteotomy (see p.3) is sometimes performed to correct deformity of the knee joint, but pain and restricted movement are the overriding reasons for considering total knee replacement.

Pain

Apart from the problems caused by disease or degeneration of the knee joint itself, pain may also sometimes be *referred* to the knee from other parts of the body, such as the hip or spine. It is therefore important that the precise cause and origin of pain in the knee joint are discovered before treatment is considered.

Osteoarthritis

Osteoarthritis is the most common form of chronic joint disease. It results from destruction and degeneration of the cartilage at the articular surfaces of joints and causes progressive joint pain and stiffness. The joints most commonly affected are the knee and hip, particularly in the elderly.

There are various types of osteoarthritis, the causes of which are not always known. It can, for example, occur following gout, infection or injury of a joint, or as a result of the death (**necrosis**) of areas of bone due to alcoholism or to the long-term use of steroids or anti-inflammatory drugs. It can also develop (most commonly in the knee) in people with haemophilia: repeated bleeding into the joint results in swelling and inflammation of the synovium, known as **synovitis**, and in the destruction of the articular cartilage.

In younger people, osteoarthritis may be the result of damage caused by fractures or previous inflammation (i.e. rheumatoid arthritis, see below). Any abnormality which puts an unusual stress on the joint (such as obesity, excessive use, for example due to strenuous physical activity, or misuse of the joint) or which increases the load (such as removal of a meniscus, see p.4), can also predispose to this disease.

In the early stages of osteoarthritis, the cartilage at the ends of the bones alters in structure and may begin to flake. Once the cartilage is lost, the surface of the bone beneath becomes exposed. By this time, the bone is likely to be more dense than normal and its exposed surface becomes worn and possibly grooved. Patches of bone may also be replaced by pockets of degenerate fibrous tissue. Small growths of cartilage known as **osteophytes** may form at the joint margins and become covered in bony material. This process of **ossification** may restrict movement of the joint.

Although the synovium is normal in the early stages of osteoarthritis, it gradually changes in character as the joint surface disintegrates, leading to synovitis (see above). Excessive synovial fluid may then escape into the joint cavity, causing swelling.

Sometimes osteoarthritis can progress rapidly while remaining painless. Because of the lack of pain, the joint continues to be used until the cartilage is destroyed and the ends of the bone are damaged. If the condition does cause pain, it may be worse in damp, cold weather and in people who are overweight and whose weight-bearing knee joints are therefore under abnormal stress. In the early stages, pain may be relieved by simple painkillers such as paracetamol. Sometimes cortisone injections may be given into the joint if the pain continues.

The management of osteoarthritis may include the use of aids such as canes or crutches to assist mobility, weight reduction by modifying the diet when necessary, stopping any inappropriate exercise which may be worsening the condition, physiotherapy to restore the strength in the muscles and the mobility of the joints as well as to help relieve pain, and drug therapy to reduce pain and inflammation.

Rheumatoid arthritis

Rheumatoid arthritis is a disease of the connective tissues which involves inflammation of several joints. It often first becomes apparent between the ages of 25 and 55, although it can affect older and younger people. It is more common in women and can cause severe crippling. The affected joints become swollen and tender, due both to synovitis and to the escape of synovial fluid into the joint cavity. The cartilage is eventually eaten away, the bones become less dense and the muscles weak and wasted. Although the disease often burns itself out in time, damage to the joints can continue and is known as **secondary osteoarthritis**.

Osteoporosis

Osteoporosis is a reduction in the density of bone which can occur as a result of decreased bone formation and/or increased bone resorption. As the bone tissue is lost, the bones become brittle and tend to fracture as a result of minor injury. Osteoporosis is an exaggeration of the natural process which occurs with age and which begins in men and women in their thirties. It can be localised or diffuse and may, for example, follow wasting away (**atrophy**) of the bones due to immobilisation or paralysis. The condition is common in post-menopausal women, suggesting an association in some cases with lack of the hormone oestrogen, production of which decreases after the menopause or following removal of the ovaries. However, the precise cause of osteoporosis is unknown.

Fractures

Bone fractures are associated with osteoporosis and are relatively common in elderly people, although they can occur at any age.

The area of bone beneath a fracture may die if its blood supply has been interrupted, possibly resulting in secondary deformity and subsequent arthritis. Hemi-arthroplasty (see p.3) may be the treatment of choice for this type of fracture.

A BRIEF HISTORY OF KNEE REPLACEMENT

Although hip replacement dates back to the early 1800s, surgery to replace the knee has only been practised for about the last 30 years.

Femoral and tibial prostheses were first developed in the early 1960s, and by the end of that decade an artificial knee was produced which was composed of a metal runner on the femoral condyle which articulated with a grooved plastic tibial component.

A couple of years later, a roller-in-a-trough femoral prosthesis was developed which depended for its stability on the integrity and tension in the ligaments on either side of the knee. Laxity of these ligaments predisposed to partial dislocation. The prosthesis was further developed a few years later to include a patellar button and an anterior femoral flange, which was subsequently grooved to constrain the patellar component and thus reduce the incidence of lateral dislocation.

In 1974, a total condylar knee was produced, the design of which has become the basis for all contemporary knee prostheses. The femoral component was symmetrical, with two identical runners joining anteriorly to form a patellar flange. The one-piece tibial component contained two cup-shaped articulating surfaces, and there was also a dome-shaped patellar component for resurfacing the patella.

Today, a wide range of prostheses is available, each with its own set of surgical instruments. Modern prostheses are manufactured in a variety of materials and are designed to meet a variety of needs. Some are symmetrical and appropriate for either knee, and some are specifically for the left or right knee. Choice of the appropriate prosthesis and its method of fixation depends to some extent on the surgeon's preference but also on various factors which are discussed in Chapter 2. Further details about the prostheses themselves, methods of fixing and the materials from which they are made are given in Chapter 3.

Tests and decisions

Most people considering total knee replacement will have had pain and possibly increasing mobility problems for some time. The possibility of surgery may be considered for anyone for whom treatment with drugs and physiotherapy has gradually become less effective, and they may be referred by their family doctor to an **orthopaedic consultant** for examination and assessment. An orthopaedic consultant is a doctor who specialises in abnormalities, diseases and injuries of the loco-motor system, i.e. all parts of the body involved in movement.

VISITING A CONSULTANT

You will receive a letter from the orthopaedic consultant giving the date and time of your appointment and any other relevant information. Although the appointment will be at a particular consultant's out-patient clinic, you may be seen by another doc-tor in the consultant's 'firm' rather than by the consultant him or herself. Details will be taken of your medical history and you will be asked about your general state of health and the causes of death of your near relatives. Movement in your knee joint will be assessed, together with your ability to walk and the presence of any associated limp. You will be asked questions about the extent to which any disability interferes with your daily activities and about the degree and pattern of pain and anything which makes it worse or better. X-rays will probably be taken of both knee joints to help diagnose the cause of the problem and to assess the existing damage.

It is important that a clear picture is built up of your general state of health and pattern of daily life so that a decision can be made about whether surgery is the right option for you. The doctor will also need to be satisfied that the risks of surgery and anaesthesia will not be increased by potential complications caused by any other illness or disability. If necessary, special tests may be arranged and an appointment may be made for you to be examined by a specialist in another branch of medicine to make sure you are fit for surgery.

Obesity

Obesity adds to the risk of general anaesthesia and can make surgery more difficult. Excess weight can also put additional strain on a replaced knee joint, possibly shortening its lifespan. Some surgeons are therefore reluctant to carry out non-emergency operations on obese patients as they consider the risks to be too great. However, starting a long, strict diet before an operation may be inadvisable and your weight will be assessed before the decision is made to go ahead with surgery and you will be given any necessary guidance by the hospital doctor.

MAKING A DECISION

There are several factors which need to be considered before a decision can be made to go ahead with surgery. As has already been mentioned, your doctor can advise you about the likely effects of surgery in your particular case, but the final decision must be made by you, bearing in mind your lifestyle, whether the pain you are suffering could be controlled by other means, and whether your expectations are realistic in terms of what you expect to be achieved by an operation. The decision about whether or not to opt for surgery is therefore very patient specific and will be influenced by the demands placed on your knee and the extent to which pain and disability affect your quality of life. Active people are likely to consider knee replacement sooner than people who are relatively sedentary. As mentioned on page 2, your motivation to comply with the demands of the rehabilitation programme must also be considered.

The following factors will have to be taken into account to assess whether surgery is the most appropriate treatment.

* *Age*. For an elderly person, will knee replacement more or less guarantee a lifetime free of pain and be unlikely to need revision? (Replaced knees have a finite life, which can be reduced by vigorous physical activity). For a younger person who hopes to lead a very active life, would it be better to postpone an operation to await further advances in technology which might enable them to do so?

* *The cause of the knee problem*.

* *The quality of bone and muscle*. As the components of a replaced knee have to be inserted into existing bone, an operation may not be feasible if the quality of your bones is generally poor. Also, poor musculature may lead to poor control of the replaced knee.

* *General physical condition*. For example, are other joints affected by arthritis which will continue to restrict your daily life or make recovery from an operation more difficult, or do you suffer from another serious medical condition which might increase the risks of surgery and anaesthesia?

* *Alternatives to total knee replacement*. Would the advantages of total knee replacement far outweigh those of other types of surgery or of non-surgical treatments?

* *Realistic expectations*. Are you likely to deal well with the period of hospitalisation involved, and to be committed to the rehabilitation process necessary post-operatively? Relatively young people who seek surgery in the hope of

continuing to take part in strenuous sporting activities should be aware that it will not realise this ambition for them. For example, it may have to be accepted that playing squash will no longer be possible, although a less vigorous sport such as golf could be taken up in its place.

* *Real need.* People who lead very sedentary lives and who spend much of their time at home may be better advised to consider non-surgical treatment to control any pain caused by a knee problem. Total knee replacement is a major operation which may be more appropriate for those wishing to resume a fairly active lifestyle.

Bilateral knee replacement If both knees are badly affected, it may be necessary to consider replacing both joints in one operation. This option would be indicated, for example, if the pain and immobility in both knee joints are so bad that replacing only one would severely restrict any attempt at rehabilitation after surgery. Severe flexion deformity may also be an indication for bilateral replacement as, if only one knee is replaced, it could adopt the deformity of the unreplaced one.

However, replacing both knee joints at the same time involves a much bigger operation and would not be considered for anyone who is frail or has contraindications such as heart or chest problems.

Once the doctor has decided that an operation would be appropriate and has discussed all the relevant factors with you, you may want to ask for time to think about it and to talk things over with your family or friends before you make a final decision. Do make sure to ask any questions you may have and do not be afraid to ask for an explanation of anything which is not clear to you. It is important that you understand exactly what is involved before consenting to surgery as ultimately the decision about whether or not to go ahead rests with *you*.

TESTS AND EXAMINATIONS

There are several tests which may need to be done before surgery which, in most cases, can be carried out at a **pre-operative assessment clinic** (see p.26). Doing these tests a few weeks or days before the operation allows time for the results to be obtained before you are admitted to hospital. If the tests reveal any infection or abnormality, the operation may have to be postponed while it is treated (see p.28).

Most people will have the pre-operative tests described below, and some may also have others specifically related to a pre-existing condition – for example a liver function test if they are known to have liver disease or damage.

* *X-rays*. A chest X-ray will be done to detect any respiratory condition which could complicate the use of a general anaesthetic or which will need to be treated before or after surgery.

    As it may be several months since an X-ray was taken of your knee at your out-patients' appointment, another may be done to detect any change in the joint which may have occurred in the intervening period.

* An *electrocardiogram*. An electrocardiogram (ECG) will be done to check that your heart is functioning normally and is healthy enough to withstand surgery. If you do have cardio-vascular problems, you may still be able to have an operation, but it is important that the surgeon and anaesthetist are aware of them so that any necessary precautions can be taken, both during and after surgery.

    As the heart beats, its muscle produces a wave of electrical energy, the pattern and size of which can be recorded via electrodes taped to the skin. A normal heart produces a distinctive pattern of electrical waves; an abnormal pattern indicates some dysfunction of the heart, such as a poor blood supply, abnormal rhythm or weak heart muscle.

During the test, electrodes will be attached to your wrists and ankles and then to the skin over your chest. The electro-cardiogram is simple and straightforward, but it is impor-tant to lie as still as possible during the few minutes it takes to do it so that electrical impulses generated by the move-ment of other muscles do not mask those from the heart. (Electrodes from a similar ECG monitor will be attached to your chest throughout the operation to make sure your heart rhythm remains normal.)

* *Blood tests*. A sample of your blood will be taken to measure its haemoglobin level. Oxygen is essential for the health and repair of the tissues of the body and for wound healing, and it is transported in the blood attached to haemoglobin. Blood will inevitably be lost during surgery, and if the level of haemoglobin is already low, it will fall even further. Therefore, if your haemoglobin level is found to be substan-tially below normal or anaemia is detected, a course of iron tablets may be prescribed to correct the problem before surgery.

The majority of people having a total knee replacement will require a blood transfusion. This is either done by filter-ing and re-infusing blood drained from the knee (see p.64) or by transfusing donor blood from another individual. It is therefore important that your blood is cross-matched so that blood of the correct group can be made available in case it is needed.

* *Urinalysis*. Urinary tract infection can give rise to post-operative infection elsewhere (with potentially serious con-sequences if it spreads to the knee). As urinary tract infec-tions can be present without causing any symptoms, a

sample of urine will be analysed to detect the presence of infective organisms. If necessary, you will be given anti-biotics to clear up any infection before the operation.

At some stage, possibly at a pre-operative assessment appointment, you will be asked several questions about any drugs you are taking, your medical history, any infection you may have, any past problems with bleeding, and if you have ever suffered any ill-effects from an anaesthetic. You will be given a thorough physical examination, including an examination of the range of movement in your affected knee joint. An inspection will probably be made of your mouth to identify any teeth which may need attention. If necessary, you will be advised to make an appointment with your dentist to have any teeth extracted *before* your operation and you will be given antibiotic cover to reduce the risk of infection. The importance of avoiding any type of infection cannot be over-emphasised. Organisms from an infec-tion anywhere in the body, however minor, can spread in the blood to a replaced knee, with potentially extremely serious consequences. The problems associated with this risk are dis-cussed in more detail on page 87.

You may also undergo one or more of the following pro-cedures.

IMAGING TECHNIQUES

Although plain X-rays usually provide adequate information about the knee, there are various imaging techniques which are sometimes used to obtain a more detailed picture of the knee joint.

Computed tomography

Computed tomography (CT) is a method of producing a series of images of the body which are interpreted by a computer. You will be asked to lie on a table which is then passed through a large hoop-shaped scanner. The various images produced by the scanner are assembled by a computer and presented as X-ray pictures of cross-sectional slices through the body.

Magnetic resonance imaging

Magnetic resonance imaging (MRI) produces images without the use of X-rays. Whereas X-rays show only bone, magnetic resonance imaging allows good depiction of the body's soft tissues and of any abnormalities within the bone marrow. Integrity of the soft tissues, such as ligaments, is essential to provide stability to the replaced joint, and magnetic resonance imaging is an excellent tool to enable an assessment of these tissues to be made. If, for example, the ligaments around the knee are lax, a prosthesis can be selected which provides additional constraint to the joint.

Like computed tomography, magnetic resonance imaging is a form of scan, providing information which is interpreted by a computer. The scanner in this case is a large, high-powered magnet contained within a scanning tunnel. Again, you will lie on a table which is passed through a tunnel as the series of scans is taken.

As the procedure involves the use of a magnet, nothing metal must be taken into the scanning tunnel, and it is unsuitable, for example, for anyone with a cardiac pacemaker. Some people find the tunnel claustrophobic and may be sedated before having this scan.

CHAPTER 3

Prostheses

Prostheses (also called components) vary according to their mode of fixation (with or without cement), the materials of which they are made, and whether they have moving or static parts. Different types may give different ranges of movement. The freedom of movement of a particular prosthesis reflects the degree of **constraint**. Some allow flexion and extension about a single fixed axis, similar to a hinge; others allow flexion and extension about a specific axis as well as some internal and external rotation. Commonly used prostheses enable the knee to bend 120 degrees or more, although a 95-degree bend is usually the maximum required during normal daily activities such as going up and down stairs and rising from a chair. Some prostheses have meniscal-bearing surfaces, with movable parts made of plastic, but most are non-meniscal and have fewer moving parts.

Prostheses are made in many different sizes to fit various-sized bones. Most are also designed to allow the option of resurfacing the underside of the knee cap. Some provide metal baseplates and wedges to which pieces of plastic of varying thicknesses can be attached for asymmetrical build-up where there is severe deformity and loss of bone. Gross deformity may require custom-made prostheses.

The selection of a suitable prosthesis will depend on factors such as your age and normal level of activity, as well as on the degree of damage and deformity of the tibia and femur. The ultimate aim of total knee replacement is to insert prostheses into the existing bone which will last indefinitely without needing to be replaced. To date, no such perfect prosthesis has been developed and thus the already wide array of options is constantly being modified and added to. A replaced knee joint may continue to function successfully for 15 years or more, but it will not last for ever. Careful consideration is therefore necessary before replacing the knee of a younger person who is likely to require revision surgery at some time in the future (see Chapter 12), and a cementless prosthesis which will preserve bone stock may be most appropriate for people in this age group.

THE TIBIAL COMPONENT

Most variation occurs in the design of the tibial component. Tibial components intended to be fixed with cement may have a prominent stem, multiple pegs or fins for attachment to the tibia. Some are made of plastic alone; some are metal backed. The metal backing may be smooth, rough surfaced or partially or entirely coated with a porous material, such as beads or fibres.

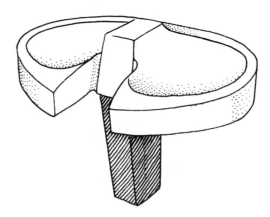

An example of a tibial component. The metal central stem is inserted into the shaft of the tibia. The surface, which articulates with the femoral component, is made of plastic.

Most tibial prostheses designed for uncemented fixation have areas of porous coating to allow bone to grow into them or bioactive coatings to encourage bone ingrowth. Others are of a press-fit design with no porous coating. They may have pegs, stems or be attached to the bone by screws.

THE FEMORAL COMPONENT

Femoral components reproduce the rounded femoral condyles of the femur. Most are designed to articulate appropriately with the plastic of the tibial component and many have an anterior flange for articulation with the knee cap. They are often fixed with small pegs or a stem.

MATERIALS

Whether or not a replaced knee is successful depends to some extent on the amount of abrasion between the articulating surfaces at the ends of the femur and tibia. Abrasion causes small

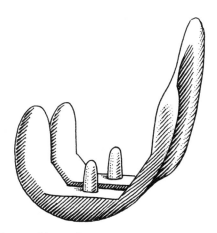

An example of a metal femoral component.

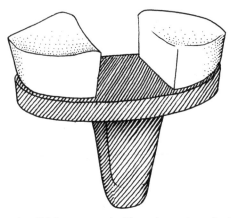

A meniscal-bearing tibial component with moving parts made of polyethylene.

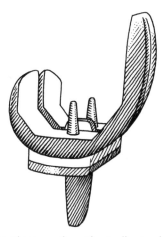

A total knee implant. This type of prosthesis allows only very little rotation of the bones.

particles to be rubbed off the surface of the prosthesis, leading to the production of **wear debris**. The wear debris causes inflammation and the bone then becomes broken down and absorbed – a process known as **osteolysis**. This can result in loosening of the components and failure of the joint. To attempt to solve this problem, many different combinations of materials have been tried over the years, and the majority of components are now made of metal – usually cobalt chrome alloy or stainless steel – and plastic in the form of high-density polyethylene. Ceramic components are rarely used for knee replacement.

* *Cobalt chrome* is a very strong metal alloy which has a high resistance to wear and to corrosion.

* *Stainless steel* is now used in the form of a new, strong, super alloy.

* *Titanium* and *titanium alloys* are strong, light metals which are very biocompatible, i.e. they allow bone to grow relatively easily onto their surface. However, in recent years there has been a movement away from using titanium as a bearing surface as it tends to be scratch and notch sensitive, properties which lead to abnormal plastic wear and sometimes to unexpected failure of the implant.

* *Polyethylene* comprises a family of plastics with similar chemical composition but different structures and thus different mechanical and wear properties. The high-density polyethylene used in today's prostheses has very good wear properties.

The fixing material

Several prostheses can be used either with or without cement, although some are specifically designed to be inserted without it. The choice depends in part on the preferred practice of the particular surgeon and on factors such as the condition of the existing bone, and on the age and activity profile of the patient.

Cement

Bone cement is formed by mixing a powder polymer with a liquid monomer. It is a brittle material which degrades with time. It is also porous and can crack if pockets of air are left in it, a problem which may be overcome by mixing it in a vacuum or centrifuging it before use.

During total knee replacement, once the ends of the tibia and femur have been prepared, cement is applied to the exposed bone ends and the prosthesis is inserted. The cement acts as a grout rather than a glue and, once set, fills the gap around the prosthesis and holds it in place. Sometimes a prosthesis is precoated with the fixing material to improve its bonding properties. *Polymethylmethacrylate* is the most commonly used fixing material but, while it has given extremely good service, there are some problems associated with its use. For example, it attains a very high temperature when setting and if it extrudes through a hole in the bone, it can cause damage to the soft tissues. It is also difficult to remove if revision surgery is required. However, at present its advantages appear to outweigh any disadvantages it may have.

Cementless fixation

Various cementless prostheses have been developed which are mainly used for younger people. However, they are currently less common in the UK than in other parts of Europe and the USA. All cementless prostheses should be made of a biocompatible material which will allow an intimate bond to form between the bone and the prosthesis.

Stability can be achieved with a good press-fit prosthesis made of biocompatible material, but many of the current cementless prostheses employ some form of biological fixation. For example, they can be coated with tiny cobalt chrome beads, titanium mesh or a bioactive substance such as *hydroxyapatite*, all of which encourage bone ingrowth, known as **osseo-integration**.

However, too much or too little stress on the bone may cause bone resorption and predispose to failure of the implant. While the short-term results of biological fixation are encouraging, its long-term performance has yet to be proven.

None of the attempts at cementless fixation has so far proved superior to the use of cement, which still remains the best option for total knee replacement. However, trials are underway to assess the effect of coating prostheses with various other biologically active materials which have a bone-like composition.

CHAPTER 4

Before your operation

You will probably be reasonably mobile by the time you are discharged from hospital, although you will have to walk with walking sticks for some weeks. However, there will still be restrictions on what you are able to do and it is a good idea to make some preparations at home before you are admitted for your operation.

PREPARING YOUR HOME

Have a look around your home to check for anything which could present a danger to you when your mobility is reduced. For example, loose rugs or mats should be taken up to avoid you slipping on them, and you should deal with any frayed edges to carpets or other potential hazards in which you could catch your foot or which could trip you up. If you have a dog or cat which tends to get under your feet, try to arrange for it to be cared for elsewhere for the first few weeks after your operation.

Although you will need someone to shop for you for at least a few days after you are discharged from hospital, you may find it useful to have a small stock of essential items before you are admitted.

PRE-OPERATIVE ASSESSMENT CLINIC

You may be given an appointment to attend a pre-operative assessment clinic some time before your operation. At many hospitals, tests are done at these clinics so that their results are available, and any necessary treatment can be given, before people are admitted for surgery. At the clinic, a doctor will explain your operation and answer any questions you may have. You should be told about the possible risks associated specifically with knee replacement surgery, such as post-operative infection (see p.87), and with operations in general, such as deep vein thrombosis (see p.85). Do make sure you understand these risks and that you are quite happy to go ahead with surgery. You may be asked to sign a **consent form** at this time, so it is particularly important that you are aware of what is involved in your operation before you do so.

Consent forms By signing a consent form you are declaring that your operation has been explained to you and that you understand what it entails, and the risks involved, and have agreed to it taking place. You are also giving your permission for the doctors to take whatever action they feel to be appropriate should some emergency occur during or after surgery, and for any necessary anaesthetic to be given to you. Do read this form carefully, and ask the doctor to explain anything you do not understand.

Total knee replacement is a major operation and, as has already been explained on page 15, a chest X-ray and electrocardiogram will be done to detect any underlying respiratory or heart disease which could complicate the use of an anaesthetic. A sample of your urine will also be taken and analysed for the presence of urinary tract infection which could lead to more serious infection after your operation. If you are found to have a urinary infection, you will probably be put on a course of anti-biotic tablets for five to seven days, at the end of which you will be told to take a further sample of urine to your family doctor. You should ring your doctor three to five days later (or as advised) to find out the results of your urine test. If the antibiotics have failed to clear the infection, it is best to ring the hospital ward or your consultant's secretary as your operation may have to be postponed for a couple of weeks to allow for further treatment. If this does occur, you will not go back on the general waiting list for surgery; every attempt should be made to do your operation within two to four weeks at most.

> **When surgery has to be postponed** It is important that medical staff are aware of *any* infection you may have (for example of your chest or urinary tract), of any other underlying disease or of the presence of a leg ulcer or cut etc., however trivial these problems may seem to you. Although it may be tempting not to mention a minor ailment – particularly if you have waited several months for your operation and cannot bear the thought of having it cancelled – it is vital that you do so. Infection can be introduced through even a small cut, with possibly devastating results if your knee were to become infected and the replaced joint had to be removed. Having to have your operation postponed for a couple of weeks because of an existing infection or other complication would be a small price to pay when compared to the unnecessarily increased risks of going ahead with anaesthesia and surgery.

Occupational therapist

An occupational therapist may be present at the pre-operative assessment clinic to explain the process of rehabilitation after your operation and to discuss any problems you might have in caring for yourself when you are discharged from hospital. Do make sure that you mention any difficulties you could face, however minor they may seem to you. Most problems can be overcome and there are various types of help available, but the more time there is to make arrangements for when you leave hospital, the better. If you do not see an occupational therapist at your pre-operative assessment appointment, you will probably do so once you are in hospital, so it may be a good idea to make a note of anything you want to discuss.

Medical social worker

If any problems are highlighted during your pre-operative assessment, a medical social worker (see p.43) can be alerted to visit you on the ward while you are in hospital to discuss the assistance which may be available when you are discharged, such as 'meals on wheels' or a home help.

Arranging transport

You should also mention at your pre-operative appointment if you will have difficulty arranging for someone to take you home when you are discharged from hospital after your operation so that nursing staff are aware that transport will need to be booked for you. However, it is better to ask a friend or relative to collect you from hospital if at all possible – and you will certainly need someone to help you at home for at least the first few days.

CHAPTER 5

Going in to hospital for an operation

Normal practice and procedures vary from hospital to hospital, and from surgeon to surgeon. The details given in this chapter about what is likely to happen when you are admitted to hospital for knee replacement surgery are therefore relatively general.

You will receive a letter from the hospital telling you the date of your operation and any other details you need to know, and may also be sent a leaflet explaining the admission procedures and what to take in with you.

If you have already attended a pre-operative assessment clinic, you are likely to be admitted to hospital on the day before your operation, otherwise you will probably be admitted a day or two beforehand for any necessary tests to be done. Once the results of these tests are known, your operation will be able to go ahead. The length of your post-operative stay in hospital will depend in part on your rate of progress, but the average is about 10 days. You will probably not be discharged until you can bend your knee at least 90 degrees, i.e. so that your calf and thigh form an inverted L shape, although the criteria for discharge vary. The practice at some hospitals, or of some surgeons, is only to discharge people once they are able to bend their knees by 90 degrees, however long that may take. At others, normal practice is to send people home after a certain number of days – providing they are well enough – even if they have obtained a lesser degree of flexion.

WHAT TO TAKE IN TO HOSPITAL

As you are likely to be in hospital for at least a week, and probably a little longer, you should give some thought to what you will need to take in with you. The following list may be helpful.

1 Nightclothes. You will be given a hospital gown to wear during your operation but will need your own nightclothes before and after it. You will also need slippers and a dressing gown. It is a good idea to have loose-fitting nightclothes, for example, for women, a nightdress which can easily be pulled up to allow them to use a bedpan and for their wounds to be checked post-operatively. Pyjama trousers will be left off altogether in the first few hours after surgery and some men find it more comfortable to wear boxer shorts instead of pyjama trousers throughout their hospital stay.

Slippers which provide good support to the feet are more comfortable and safer than floppy slippers or mules. Your leg is likely to be swollen after your operation and this swelling, together with the additional bulk of anti-embolism stockings (see p.40), may make it impossible to get your feet into tight-fitting or new and unworn slippers.

2 Clothes. There is no reason why you should continue to wear your nightclothes once you are up and mobile after your operation. Shoes should provide good support to your feet without being tight, and should be flat or have a low heel. High-heeled shoes are inappropriate and potentially dangerous when your are regaining mobility after surgery.

Restrictive clothing may impair the circulation of a swollen limb, and therefore any tight-fitting clothes, such as panty girdles or jeans, should be avoided. They will also be uncomfortable and difficult to get on and off in the first few days after surgery.

You will probably be able to wear your own underpants

under your hospital gown during your operation, provided they are made entirely of cotton: synthetic materials can cause a build-up of static when electrical equipment is used during surgery. Alternatively, you can wear paper, disposable underpants, which may be available on the ward. The elastic around the legs of your underpants should be loose.

3   *Towel and washing things.*

4   *Walking aids/surgical shoes.* You should take in to hospital any walking aids you already use as they may need to be repaired or changed to suit your gait after surgery. People who have suffered pain and disability prior to knee replacement surgery develop an abnormal gait which will have to be corrected post-operatively. It is therefore important that their walking aids are adapted to suit a more normal way of walking.

If you have been wearing surgical or specially adapted shoes, you should also take these in to hospital with you in case any alterations need to be made to them.

5   *Money, jewellery etc.* A *small* amount of money may be useful for newspapers and the telephone. Large sums of money, handbags, wallets and jewellery should not be taken into hospital as these may have to be kept in an unlocked cabinet by your bed. Any valuables or large sums of money you have to take with you should be given to the ward sister for safe keeping when you are admitted. You will be given a receipt listing each item, which you should keep safe so that you can collect your possessions when you are discharged. However, hospital authorities strongly discourage people from bringing anything of great value with them unless absolutely necessary. It is better to make arrangements for any valuables you do not wish to leave at home to be looked after by a relative or friend while you are in hospital.

6   *Books, magazines, puzzles etc.* There will inevitably be periods of waiting between visits from medical staff before your operation, and you may want something to occupy you during this time as well as post-operatively.

7   *Drugs you are already taking.* Once your admission has been arranged, your family doctor will have been asked to fill in a form stating all the drugs you are taking and their doses. You may be asked to take your drugs with you when you are admitted to hospital so that their dosages can be checked and so that you can continue to be given any which are necessary. All your drugs will be kept for you during your stay as you must only take those which are given to you by medical staff. They should, however, be returned to you before you leave.

8   *Admission letter.* You should take with you the admission letter sent to you from the hospital.

Wedding rings Wedding rings, or any other rings which are very precious to you or which cannot be removed, will be covered with adhesive tape before your operation. This is to prevent the metal causing burns during the process of **electrocautery** (or **diathermy**) which is used to control bleeding during surgery. In electrocautery, an electric current heats the tip of an instrument which is used to shrivel and seal the little blood vessels and stop them bleeding.

HOSPITAL STAFF

The ward of a hospital is a busy place and can seem rather confusing and frightening. It may help to have an idea of the different medical staff you are likely to meet, and the jobs they do.

Nurses

The uniforms worn to distinguish nurses of different ranks will vary from hospital to hospital, but all nurses wear badges which state clearly their name and sometimes their grade. There are, of course, both male and female nurses, although women are still in the majority. The nursing grades are as follows.

1   The most senior nurse on the ward is the *ward sister* or *ward manager*. Each ward will have one ward sister who will be very experienced and able to answer any questions you may have. The ward sister has 24-hour a day responsibility for all the staff and patients on at least one ward, for the day-to-day running of the ward, standards of care etc., and is ultimately responsible for the ward even when not on duty. She will be a registered nurse (RN) or a registered general nurse (RGN), who has usually been qualified for at least five years. Ward sisters may wear a uniform of a single colour, often dark blue.

   The male equivalent of the ward sister is a *charge nurse*, whose rank will be clearly displayed on his name badge. Charge nurses wear a white tunic.

2   When the ward sister is not on duty, there may be a *senior staff nurse* or a *team leader* of another grade in charge. The senior staff nurse is deputy to, and works closely with, the ward sister. Like the ward sister, this nurse will be very experienced.

3   Each ward may have several *staff nurses*. They may be newly qualified or may have several years' experience, and will take charge of the ward when both the ward sister and senior staff nurse are unavailable. There are different grades of staff nurse, distinguished by different coloured belts, epaulettes, uniforms or, more rarely nowadays, hats.

The more junior staff nurses, who are often in their first or second post since qualifying, are less involved in ward management, and are therefore able to work closely with the patients.

4   *Enrolled nurses* have undergone two years of training. They are gradually being replaced and can now undergo a training programme to become staff nurses with the qualification RGN. However, there are still many enrolled nurses working on hospital wards who are very experienced and sometimes team leaders (see above).

5   As student nurses now spend more time in college and less on the wards of hospitals, *health care assistants* (HCAs) are being brought in to take their place. These are unqualified nurses who have undergone six months' training on day release while working on a ward and who have then been assessed for a National Vocational Qualification (NVQ) by senior nurses. Health care assistants are able to carry out all basic nursing duties except for the dispensing of drugs. They are supervised at all times by a qualified nurse.

6   The ward may also have several *nursing auxiliaries* who are present to deal with any non-medical jobs and to help with the basic care of patients such as making beds, serving tea, and putting away linen etc. Although nursing auxiliaries are not trained nurses, some are very experienced and have acquired greater responsibility.

7   Student nurses – *diploma nursing students* or *Project* 2000 *students* – are unpaid and allocated to the wards at various stages during their college-based training. They are mainly involved in observing and carrying out limited clinical tasks. In their last term before they qualify, they will be rostered on to nursing shifts and be part of a ward team.

Doctors

Each consultant surgeon in a hospital may head a team of doctors of different ranks, sometimes known as a 'firm'. You may meet some or all of them. These doctors can, of course, be men or women.

1 The *consultant surgeon* holds the ultimate responsibility for all the patients on the operating list, and for the work of all the staff in the 'firm'. Consultants have at least 10 to 15 years' experience as surgeons.

   Unless you are being treated privately (see Chapter 13), you may see the consultant who is responsible for your care at your first out-patient appointment and possibly during a ward round after your operation. Otherwise, you are likely to be seen by a registrar (see below). You should be visited on the ward before your operation by whichever surgeon is to perform it.

2 The *senior registrar* is an experienced surgeon who has completed several years of training and will soon be appointed to a consultant post. (This grade of surgeon is soon to be changed.)

3 Your operation may be performed by a *registrar* rather than by a consultant surgeon or senior registrar. Registrars have trained as surgeons for at least two or three years and are able to carry out some surgery alone, assisting the consultant or being assisted by the consultant on more difficult operations.

4 Some hospitals employ *clinical assistants* as surgeons. These are often very experienced surgeons who, for personal or family reasons, are not able to work full time.

5 You may be examined before your operation by a *senior house officer* (SHO) or by a house surgeon (see below). Senior

house officers have been qualified doctors for between one and five years, and are gaining further experience in hospital before becoming surgical registrars or specialising in another branch of medicine.

6   A *house surgeon* (or *house officer*) is likely to be directly concerned with your care both before and after your operation, taking notes of your medical history and arranging for any necessary pre-operative investigations to be done, such as a blood count, chest X-ray and electrocardiogram. House officers are qualified doctors who have completed at least five years of undergraduate training and are working for a further year in hospital before becoming fully registered. Although house officers do not perform surgery on their own, they may assist the surgeon in the operating theatre.

Anaesthetists are doctors who have been trained in the administration of drugs which cause loss of sensation or consciousness, or both (anaesthetics), and those which block feelings of pain (analgesics). An anaesthetist may visit you before your operation to discuss any relevant details, such as any anaesthetics you have had in the past and any drugs you may be taking (see Chapter 6), and will be present throughout your operation.

ADMISSION TO THE WARD

When you arrive at the hospital, you should report to the main reception desk with your admission letter. The staff there will check your details and tell you which ward to go to. Once on the ward, the ward clerk or a nurse will deal with the clerical side of your admission, filling in the necessary forms with you. You will then be shown to your bed and told of any ward details such as meal times, where to find the toilets, day room etc.

In Britain, the 'Named Nurse Initiative' was introduced under the Government's Patients' Charter. In a National Health Service

(NHS) hospital, each patient is allocated a **named nurse** who is responsible for planning that patient's nursing care throughout their stay. The ward sister will, of course, still be informed of all aspects of your care, and will be able to discuss it with you or your relatives.

Your named nurse will admit you to the ward, look after you during your stay, and co-ordinate your discharge when the time comes. Other nurses will be allocated from the team for other working shifts. The idea is for people to be identified as individuals who are known to at least one nurse on each shift and who are involved in their own care. To this end, you may be asked to help your nurse draw up a care plan when you are admitted to the ward. You should tell the nurse of any ailments, preferences or dislikes you have, for example if you prefer to sleep with several pillows or if there are certain foods you do not want.

Your nurse's name may be displayed above your bed or on your bedside locker so that your relatives and other nursing and medical staff know who to talk to about your care. Your care plan may be kept at the bottom of your bed, but wherever it is, it is available for you to read. Nursing staff may tick off a checklist as they carry out the various procedures and will update the care plan with you as the need arises.

Questionnaires Apart from being involved in research of one type or another, hospital staff are always attempting to improve the care they offer. Therefore, on admission to hospital you may be given a questionnaire to fill in before you leave, giving details of the positive and negative aspects of your hospital stay. You will not be asked to sign the form, and can therefore feel free to be honest in your answers without the fear of causing offence. It is very helpful to hospital staff to receive feedback from their patients so that they can be sure they are providing the right service in the right way, and you should try to complete any questionnaire you are given if at all possible.

The nurse will measure your blood pressure, temperature and pulse. A sample of your urine may be taken for analysis and you may be weighed if the anaesthetist needs to know your weight to calculate the dose of anaesthetic you require.

Do tell a nurse if you have any problems or if you are anxious about *any* aspect of your hospital stay.

Clinical trials To be able to improve the treatment given to people, new therapies need to be tested, and currently used treatment regimes need to be tried in different ways. Therefore you may be asked to take part in a clinical trial to compare a new treatment with an existing one.

The details of any trial will be explained to you, and you should make sure you fully understand what is entailed before you make a decision. Once you understand the implications of the trial, and if you agree to be included, you will be asked to sign a consent form. You are under no obligation to take part in a clinical trial and, if you refuse, the quality of the treatment you receive will not be affected in any way.

THROMBOSIS PREVENTION

Normally, the activity of the muscles in the legs helps to keep the blood moving through them. During long periods of bed rest or anaesthesia, these muscles are inactive and the circulation of blood in the legs slows down. A blood clot – known as a **thrombus** – is thus more likely to form and can block the passage of blood through the vein, causing a **thrombosis** (see p.85). If a piece of the blood clot breaks off, it forms an **embolus** which may travel through the circulation and lodge in a vital organ such as the lung, causing a **pulmonary embolism**, with serious consequences.

There are various precautions which can be taken to reduce the risk of a thrombosis developing.

Anti-embolism stockings

Once you are settled on the ward, a nurse will measure your legs for anti-embolism stockings (often called TEDS – **t**hrombo-**e**mbolic **d**eterrent **s**tockings). These stockings are used routinely in some hospitals, and are invariably worn by anyone having a knee replacement operation and whose mobility will be limited to some degree for several weeks. They improve the return of blood to the heart and are thought to help prevent blood clots forming in the deep veins of the legs.

Once you have had a bath or shower (see p.45) and are getting ready to leave the ward for your operation, an anti-embolism stocking will probably be put on the leg which is not being operated on. A stocking will be put on the operated leg 48 to 72 hours after your operation when the pressure bandage is removed from your knee (see p.61). You will have to wear both stockings for about six weeks. When necessary, they should be washed during the day while you are mobile and dried to wear again at night, when the risk of thrombosis is greater. They should never be dried over direct heat, such as on a radiator, as it will reduce their elasticity and therefore their effectiveness.

Foot pumps

You may be given special boots to wear while you are in bed after your operation. These boots, which are designed to reduce the risk of deep vein thrombosis, are made of a soft, foam-like material and attached to a foot pump at the end of the bed. A pocket under each foot systematically inflates and deflates, assisting the circulation of blood in the legs. If you are given foot pumps, they will probably be kept on whenever you are in bed throughout your stay in hospital. You will be helped to take them off and put them on again when you want to get out of and into bed. Although the value of these foot pumps is still being assessed, they are already used routinely in some hospitals.

Heparin injections

You may also be given injections of low-dose heparin throughout your stay in hospital to reduce the risk of blood clots forming. Heparin is an anticoagulant which occurs naturally in the body, thinning the blood and helping to prevent it from clotting. (Higher doses of heparin, or of a similar substance called warfarin, can be given to treat a blood clot once it has developed.) Heparin injections are not given routinely in all hospitals, but they are invariably necessary for anyone at particular risk of thrombosis.

WARD VISIT BY A DOCTOR

As has already been mentioned, a house surgeon or senior house officer will visit you on the ward before your operation to take details of your medical history – including any allergies you may have and any drugs you are taking – and to examine you. Your family doctor may have already filled in a form giving the names and dosages of any drugs you have been prescribed, and you should have been told what to do about these. Do not forget to tell the hospital doctor of any other drugs you have been taking which your family doctor may not be aware of, such as vitamin supplements, cough medicines, aspirins etc., which are available from a pharmacy without the need for a prescription.

A medical examination will be carried out to detect any illness or infection you may have which could complicate the use of a general anaesthetic. You may also have a chest X-ray, an electrocardiogram, a urine test and a blood test, even if you have already had these at a pre-operative assessment clinic. If you have rheumatoid arthritis, an X-ray may be taken of your neck to make sure you have sufficient movement in it to enable the anaesthetist to insert a tube through your mouth during anaesthesia.

The surgeon who is to perform your operation may also visit you on the ward to check that all is well. If you have not already done so, you will be asked to sign a consent form (see p.27).

WARD VISIT BY AN ANAESTHETIST

An anaesthetist will probably come to see you before your operation to discuss anything that may be relevant to the choice of anaesthetic given to you. Do make sure that you mention any aspect of your anaesthesia which causes you concern so that the anaesthetist can explain things to you and put your mind at rest. For example, many people are anxious about anaesthetics being administered through a face mask. Although face masks are now not normally used until patients are sedated, it is worth mentioning this fear so that your anaesthetist is aware of it and can reassure you.

Pre-medication

Anaesthetics have improved considerably during the last few years, and a 'pre-med.' is now not always given routinely. However, if you enter hospital the day before your operation and think that you will be too anxious to sleep that night, do ask the house surgeon or senior house officer for something to help you.

Sometimes spinal or epidural anaesthetics (see Chapter 6) are injected in the operating theatre while the patient is sitting on the edge of the operating table, supported by a nurse. In these cases, sedation with a pre-med. is not appropriate as patients need to be alert and able to comply with simple instructions while the injection is administered. Some people are upset if they expect to have a pre-med. and are told they cannot have one, and it is best to be prepared in advance for this possibility.

If you are having a pre-med., it will be given to you an hour or two before your operation to sedate you. If it is routine practice in your hospital for everyone to have a pre-med., do tell the anaesthetist if you prefer to do without one.

False teeth

You should tell the anaesthetist if you have any false teeth or dental bridges as these will have to be removed before you go into the operating theatre. A broken or loose tooth can be inhaled into the lungs during surgery. You should also point out any teeth which are crowned. In some hospitals people are able to wear their false teeth until they reach the operating theatre rather than having to take them out on the ward.

WARD VISITS BY OTHER STAFF

It is sometimes routine practice for operating theatre staff to visit people on the ward before their operations to explain theatre procedures and equipment to them. You may also be introduced to a nurse from the recovery room, possibly when you are taken to the operating theatre. These visits are made in an attempt to reduce some of the anxiety associated with surgery by introducing people to the nurses who will care for them during and immediately after their operation.

Medical social workers

If any problems arise at home during your stay in hospital, or if you are concerned about being able to manage on your own once you are discharged, you can ask to talk to a medical social worker. Medical social workers work in close partnership with other medical staff in the hospital and are able to give advice and practical support. If necessary, you may be kept in hospital a little longer than normal until nursing staff are happy that you will be able to manage or that arrangements have been made to help you once you are at home.

It is important that enough time is allowed to make arrangements for any necessary assistance once you leave hospital, and you should therefore make known any potential problems as soon as possible, ideally at your pre-operative assessment appointment.

Physiotherapists

A physiotherapist is someone who is trained to assist patients to rehabilitate following illness, injury or deformity. You may have been referred to a physiotherapist some time before your operation if you needed special treatment such as hydrotherapy for a particular problem.

A physiotherapist may visit you on the ward before your operation to assess your mobility and any problems you have, such as deformity or loss of use of other joints due, for example, to rheumatoid arthritis, which could affect the post-operative exercises you are able to do, or the way you do them. This visit is useful in that it allows the physiotherapist to plan an exercise routine tailored to your individual needs.

During the physiotherapist's visit, you may also be shown how to do some simple exercises immediately after your operation, such as ankle movements to assist your circulation while you are immobile in bed (see p.63). The physiotherapist may ask you to try to lift your bottom off the bed by pushing yourself up using your good leg. The ability to do this will enable you to change your position in bed after your operation, to make yourself more comfortable and to help to avoid pressure sores. If you cannot change your position in this way, a special **monkey pole** may be attached above your bed for you to hold onto.

The physiotherapist will discuss with you the importance of deep breathing to help reduce the risk of chest problems post-operatively, and may show you some breathing exercises. He or she will probably already be aware of any specific problems you have which may affect your post-operative rehabilitation, and may talk to you about these. Your rehabilitation programme will also be explained to you.

PREPARING FOR SURGERY

There are several routine procedures which will take place in the hours before your operation.

'Nil by mouth'

This is a term which means that neither food nor drink must be swallowed. In order to prevent vomiting and the risk of choking on your vomit while you are anaesthetised, you may be told not to eat or drink anything for four to six hours before your operation, although you will be able to have a few sips of water with any tablets you need to take. Even people having an epidural or spinal anaesthetic will be given some sort of sedation during their operation, and it is always possible that surgery started with a spinal or epidural anaesthetic may have to be completed using general anaesthesia. Therefore, whatever type of anaesthetic you are due to have, you will be 'nil by mouth' in the preceding hours, although some anaesthetists now allow their patients to drink clear fluids up to three hours pre-operatively.

Bathing

You may be told to have a bath or shower a couple of hours or more before your operation, either during the morning of the same day or the night before. You can use ordinary soap and water but should not use deodorant, talcum powder, nail varnish, perfume etc.

Shaving

The operation site is unlikely to be shaved before knee surgery. Although this used to be routine practice, it is now thought that shaving has the potential to increase the risk of infection post-operatively.

Smoking

If you are a heavy smoker and have not been able to cut down or stop altogether, you will be advised not to smoke in the hours before your operation. It is, of course, much better to stop smoking some months before surgery, and some surgeons will not perform non-emergency operations on heavy smokers. The carbon monoxide contained in cigarette smoke poisons the blood by replacing some of the oxygen which is carried in it and which is vital to processes such as wound healing. Smoking also increases the risk of chest infection post-operatively.

Waiting

As already mentioned, you are likely to be admitted to hospital at least the day before your operation so that any necessary tests and examinations can be done and their results received and so that all the staff mentioned above can visit you on the ward.

Occasionally surgery has to be cancelled at the last moment because an emergency has arisen and an earlier operation has taken longer than expected or has met with complications. If this does occur, you may be sent home and called again at the earliest opportunity. Although this would obviously be distressing, do try not to get upset. Other operations taking place on the same day may be more urgent than yours and be unable to be postponed. In the UK, under the terms of the Patients' Charter, a cancelled operation must be done within one month, and the medical staff will certainly make every effort to do yours as soon as possible.

You will probably be given only an approximate time of day for your operation.

Leaving the ward for your operation

Before being taken from the ward to the anaesthetic room or operating theatre, the knee to be operated on will be marked with a felt-tip pen. You may be asked several times by different medical staff – possibly including the surgeon – which knee joint is to be replaced. Do not be worried by this question; it does not mean that they do not know! Repeated checks of this sort help to avoid mistakes being made, which are possible when so many operations are done each day in a large and busy hospital.

You will be given a hospital operating gown to wear; a plastic-covered bracelet bearing your name and an identifying hospital number will be attached to one or each of your wrists; and an anti-embolism stocking will be put on your 'good' leg. You will then leave the ward on a hospital trolley.

If you wear a hearing aid, it is unlikely to have to be removed until you are asleep, and will probably be put back when you are in the recovery room after your operation.

The anaesthetic room

In the anaesthetic room, a small tube called a **cannula** will be inserted into a vein in the back of your hand. The cannula will be kept in place throughout the operation to provide a channel for the administration of drugs. The anaesthetic will probably be administered in the anaesthetic room, although it may be given in the operating theatre itself. A general anaesthetic will take effect within seconds, a spinal or epidural anaesthetic within a matter of minutes. Once the anaesthetist is satisfied that you are properly anaesthetised, you are ready for your operation.

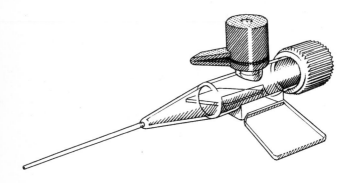

A cannula. The cannula is inserted into a vein in the back of the hand and drugs are administered through it during surgery.

CHAPTER 6

Anaesthesia and pain relief

This chapter describes the different anaesthetics used for knee replacement operations. The anaesthetic chosen will depend on various factors, including the type of operation you are having and the normal practice of your anaesthetist. It may be possible for your own preferences to be taken into account, if you have any, so do discuss them with the anaesthetist during the ward visit.

REGIONAL ANAESTHESIA

Regional anaesthesia is sometimes used, usually in combination with a sedative to put you to sleep. It is a form of local anaesthesia for which the anaesthetic drug is contained within a specific area of the body. You may be given one of two types, either a spinal or an epidural. Sometimes a tracheal tube is inserted to keep the airways open, in which case you may also be given a very light general anaesthetic to enable the tube to be passed down your throat.

Spinal anaesthesia

For a spinal anaesthetic, the drug is injected between the vertebrae of the spine into the space around the nerves in the back. It causes numbness in the legs and groin which lasts for between one and a half and three hours, or longer in older people. The anaesthetic takes effect within about five minutes, causing the legs and lower body to become numb and heavy. Spread of the drug can be controlled within the desired area by the addition of glucose to make it heavier and by appropriate positioning of your body during the operation.

Spinal anaesthetics induce profound muscle relaxation and can be used in low doses, thus avoiding any complications of toxicity. However, they can cause headaches and have a limited duration of action.

Epidural anaesthesia

Epidural anaesthesia is similar to spinal anaesthesia and is sometimes used for knee operations. The anaesthetic drug is injected into the back but, unlike for a spinal anaesthetic, the needle does not penetrate the membrane around the spinal cord (the **dura**). The effects of an epidural last longer than those of a spinal anaesthetic and epidurals can therefore provide pain relief for a period after surgery.

A small tube called a **catheter** is inserted into the back and left in place throughout the operation so that additional doses of the drug can be introduced as required. The catheter is sometimes retained for a day or two after surgery so that pain-killing drugs can be administered through it.

Epidural anaesthetics take 15 minutes or more to have an effect.

GENERAL ANAESTHESIA

Most knee replacement operations are done using general anaesthesia. A general anaesthetic will put you to sleep so that you have no feeling in any part of your body. It may be an **intravenous anaesthetic**, injected into a vein in your hand or arm through a plastic tube, or an **inhalational anaesthetic** in the form of a gas which you breathe in. In fact, both types are normally used, although you will probably only be aware of the injection which sends you off to sleep.

If you are having a general anaesthetic, you may be visited on the ward by an anaesthetist before your operation (see p.42). The main reason for this visit is to decide what type of anaesthesia would be safest for you. It also gives you the opportunity to discuss any problems or worries you may have. The anaesthetist will ask you several questions about any anaesthetics you have had before, any drugs you are taking, and about your general health. It is important that you answer these questions as fully as possible. You should also mention to the anaesthetist if you have any false or crowned teeth (see p.43).

If you have had problems in the past such as an allergy to a particular anaesthetic, it will be helpful if you know the name of the drug concerned and/or the hospital where the operation was carried out. The appropriate records can then be checked to make sure another type of anaesthetic is used. You should also tell the anaesthetist if you know of any member of your family who has reacted against a particular drug, as you may have the same problem.

During your operation

If you are having a general anaesthetic, several different types of drugs will be given to you during your operation:

* *induction agents* to bring on sleep;

* *maintenance agents* to keep you asleep;

* *analgesics* to stop you feeling pain after the operation;

* *anti-emetics* to help stop you feeling sick after the operation;

* *muscle relaxants*.

Analgesics and anti-emetics are also given post-operatively as required.

When the operation is over, the anaesthetist will stop giving you the drugs that were keeping you asleep, and you will be taken to a recovery room (see p.54).

Side-effects of general anaesthesia

There are some side-effects related to the use of general anaesthetics, but these are usually minor and do not last very long. The most common are nausea and vomiting. You may also have a sore throat after your operation, possibly due to the 'dry' anaesthetic gases used to keep you asleep during surgery, or to the tube which may have been placed in your throat to maintain an airway and help you to breathe. Whatever the reason, any soreness usually disappears after two or three days and can be eased by simple painkillers. The muscle relaxants used during anaesthesia can cause muscle aches and pains, which should improve within about 48 hours.

Risks of general anaesthesia

Some people are afraid of being put to sleep by a general anaesthetic, but the risk is small. Advances in anaesthesia over the past few years have been tremendous. Although complications still occasionally occur and, very rarely, people do suffer brain damage or even die during surgery – risks which do need to be borne in mind – you are far more likely to be killed in a road accident than to suffer any serious ill-effect from the use of an anaesthetic.

Careful consideration will be given by the surgeon and anaesthetist to your general state of health and all other relevant factors before deciding to go ahead with your operation and anaesthesia. People with certain medical conditions, such as serious heart or lung disease, may not be given general anaesthetics as they are potentially at greater risk. However, if you are worried about any risks involved, do discuss your concerns with the anaesthetist.

OTHER MEDICATION

The anaesthetist will explain about other tablets and drugs which may be required before your operation. You may be given the option of having a 'pre-med.', usually in the form of tablets given one to two hours before surgery. If you are anxious about your operation, you may wish to ask for a 'pre-med.' if their use is not routine in your hospital.

The anaesthetist will also explain about any antibiotics or anticoagulants (blood-thinning drugs) you may require. Drugs which you normally take, such as diuretics ('water tablets') or drugs to reduce high blood pressure, may also be continued but you must only take those which are given to you by medical staff.

BEFORE YOUR OPERATION

You will probably be told not to have anything to eat or drink for about six hours before your operation ('nil by mouth', see p.45). If you are having a 'pre-med.', it may be given to you while you are still on the ward, and you will soon begin to feel sleepy. There is no need to be alarmed: the 'pre-med.' is not an anaesthetic itself, it is only to relax you and stop you feeling anxious.

When you are taken from the ward, you may go first to the anaesthetic room or straight to the operating theatre to be given your anaesthetic. The anaesthetist, or an assistant, will fit some monitoring devices to watch over you while you are asleep. These may include a little probe which goes on your finger to measure the amount of oxygen in your blood, an electrocardiogram (ECG) to observe your heart beat (see p.15), and a cuff around your arm to measure your blood pressure. Once the anaesthetist is happy with the readings from these monitors, the anaesthesia will start.

If you are having a general anaesthetic, a cannula will be put into a vein in the back of your hand or arm (see p.48), and the anaesthetic drugs will be introduced into your body through it. Once the anaesthetic has been injected, you will fall asleep within seconds. The drug which makes you go to sleep may sting a little as it enters the vein from the cannula, but this feeling does not last long.

For a spinal or epidural anaesthetic, you will be asked to sit on the edge of the bed or trolley or to lie on your side while the drug is injected into your back.

The anaesthetist will remain with you throughout the operation to make sure you are asleep and that the function of your heart and lungs is satisfactory.

THE RECOVERY ROOM

When your operation is over, you will be taken to the recovery room. The nurses in the recovery room are specially trained to care for patients coming round from anaesthetics after an operation. You will stay in this room, still watched over by monitoring equipment, until you are fully awake and ready to be returned to your own ward.

If you are in any pain when you wake up, the staff in the recovery room will be able to give you something to relieve it. This can be an injection either through the cannula which is already in place or directly into your arm or buttock. If you have had an epidural anaesthetic, the catheter will probably still be in your back so that pain-killing drugs can be introduced through it as required.

PAIN RELIEF

The amount of pain or discomfort experienced after any operation varies from person to person, and of course also depends on the extent of the surgery involved.

The house surgeon and nurses on your ward will be able to give you analgesics for any pain. However, if these are not enough, do ask the anaesthetist or ward staff for something more effective. Knee surgery is painful, and the pain must be controlled adequately to enable you to do the necessary post-operative exercises.

If you have had an epidural anaesthetic, morphine can be introduced through the catheter already in place in your back. Otherwise, you will probably be given injections of morphine every two to three hours for at least the first six hours after your operation.

Patient-controlled analgesia

In some hospitals, patient-controlled analgesia (PCA) may be offered after a knee operation, but PCA machines are expensive and may not be available for all patients. The PCA technique has been designed to allow patients themselves to control the amount of analgesic they receive. With the exception of epidural analgesia, which is particularly effective in the first 48 hours or so after knee surgery, PCA is generally a better way of providing pain relief than most of the conventional forms.

If a PCA machine is available, you will be given clear instructions about how to use it. It is basically a pump which delivers a pain-killing drug into your body each time you press a button. It is programmed to allow you only a safe limit of the drug, which is usually delivered via a cannula in a vein in your hand or arm. When you press the button, your pain should start to reduce within five to ten minutes. If it does not do so, press the button again. As the machine has a built-in safety control to prevent you receiving too much of the drug, you can press the button as often as you like. However, it is important that you do not let anyone else use your machine as doing so would remove the safety feature. If, despite pressing the button several times, your pain is not being relieved, tell a nurse or doctor as it may be possible for the machine to be reset to deliver a stronger dose of the drug.

A nurse or doctor will inspect the counter on your machine at regular intervals to see how many times you have pressed the button and how much analgesic drug you have received. Once it is clear that you are reducing the amount of drug you need, and therefore your pain is improving, the machine setting will be changed to deliver a lower dose at each press of the button. Patient-controlled analgesia (or analgesic injections) can nor-mally be replaced by analgesic tablets after 24 to 48 hours.

CHAPTER 7

The operation

This chapter explains the surgical procedures involved in total knee replacement. The details are the same for hemi-arthroplasty, with the exception that only half the joint is removed and replaced by prostheses.

TOTAL KNEE REPLACEMENT

The operation is normally carried out under a general anaesthetic or using a spinal anaesthetic and sedative. Once the anaesthetic has taken effect, you will be placed on the operating table with your knee flexed and your foot supported on a sandbag.

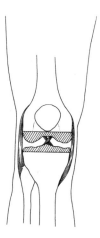

The knee joint. The shaded areas of the femur and tibia are cut away before the prostheses are inserted.

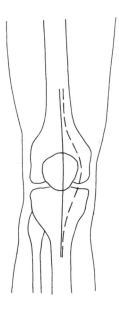

Deep incision. The line of a typical incision made in the skin (solid line) and in the muscle and capsule (dashed line) during total knee replacement.

A tourniquet is placed around the thigh to reduce blood loss during the operation, and an incision about 20 cm (8 inches) long is usually made in the midline of the knee. However, if you have had previous knee surgery and there are scars on the inside of your knee, the line of incision will deviate from the midline to pass through these pre-existing scars. The soft tissues beneath the skin (the joint capsule and synovium) are then incised, the incision being continued up towards the hip for about 5 cm (approximately 2 inches), through the dense tendon of the quadriceps muscle. The knee cap is then dislocated laterally.

Using a range of highly sophisticated surgical instruments, the upper end of the tibia and the lower end of the femur are cut

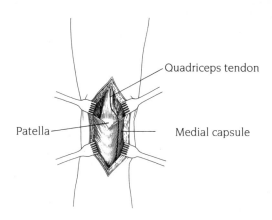

Deep incision through the tendon of the quadriceps muscle and the medial capsule.

away (**resected**). The tibia is cut parallel to the floor, and the femur is cut at an angle which maintains the normal alignment of the leg.

Specially designed instruments are used to sculpt the end of the femur to accept the metal femoral prosthesis, and a trial component is applied to the femur. The cut surface of the upper end of the tibia is prepared to accept the baseplate of the tibial prosthesis. Once the baseplate is in place, plastic (which will provide the bearing surface) is added to it to bridge the gap beween the two prostheses. The plastic should be of suitable thickness to tension the soft tissues around the knee appropriately. The knee is then restored to its normal position (**reduced**), and the surgeon puts it through a range of movement and tests it for stability.

If the patella is going to be resurfaced, its undersurface is cut away, fixation holes are prepared using a jig, and a plastic trial component is inserted. The patella is then reduced and the knee is again flexed to ensure that it runs centrally. If there is a tendency for the patella to dislocate, the tissues on the outer aspect of the knee are progressively released until the patella tracks centrally.

All the trial components are then removed, the bone is cleaned and dried, and the prostheses are cemented into position. Care is taken to remove all the cement which extrudes from the fixation points.

The wound is closed in layers, with two suction drains being left inside, and a compression bandage is applied to the knee. You will then be taken to the recovery room to come round from the anaesthetic.

CHAPTER 8

After your operation: in hospital

When you come round from the anaesthetic, you will be taken from the recovery room back to your hospital ward. You may have been put back onto your own bed in the operating theatre while still anaesthetised so that you are subjected to as little 'manhandling' as possible.

The compression bandage put around your knee at the end of the operation will be left in place for 48 to 72 hours and will then be replaced with an anti-embolism stocking (see p.40). You will be virtually unable to bend your leg while the compression bandage is on.

You will be encouraged (and assisted) to become mobile again as soon as possible, and will probably be helped to get out of bed for the first time a couple of days after your operation. Normal practice varies from hospital to hospital as well as from surgeon to surgeon, and the specific advice given to you by medical staff will depend on these factors as well as on your particular requirements. This chapter therefore gives a general idea of what to expect during your post-operative hospital stay. Always make sure you understand any advice you are given. Hospital staff are aware of the difficulty of absorbing information in the days following an operation and should be happy to repeat any explanations as often as necessary.

You may be given oxygen via a face mask immediately after your operation to assist wound healing if your breathing is shallow. Deep breathing and coughing will help to keep your lungs supplied with oxygen and clear of sputum. If you are at particular risk of chest infection or have a respiratory complaint, a physiotherapist will advise you about some exercises to do.

Physiotherapists play a significant part in the rehabilitation of people following knee replacement surgery. Your physiotherapist will probably have talked to you before your operation and will visit you on the ward the day after it. Chapter 9 deals in more detail with the role of the physiotherapist and with the exercises you will need to do to give yourself the best chance of regaining as much mobility as possible in your knee.

Four or five days after your operation, when you are able to get out of bed and have regained some mobility, an occupational therapist will also visit you on the ward to see how you are managing. Apart from making sure you are able to get out of bed, wash and dress yourself, the occupational therapist will help you to deal with any problems which may arise. He or she may visit you two or three times while you are in hospital to discuss ways of managing more easily when you return home. Do ask about anything which worries you or which you are not sure you will be able to do. Also, if your relatives have any concerns, they can ask to talk to your occupational therapist, either when they visit you in hospital or by telephone.

PAIN RELIEF

For the first few hours after your operation, you will be given morphine for pain relief – by injection, epidural or PCA machine (see p.55). As morphine can induce sickness, you will also have anti-emetic injections to help counteract this effect. After this, you will be able to take regular analgesic tablets, which you are likely to need to continue taking for several weeks to enable you to do the necessary exercises. While in hospital, do tell a doctor or nurse if your pain is not being controlled as it may be possible to give you something stronger.

THROMBOSIS PREVENTION

Blood clots are most common about two days after knee surgery, although they can develop anytime up to three weeks or later.

You will continue to wear anti-embolism stockings (see p.40) throughout your stay in hospital and possibly for up to six weeks until the risk of deep vein thrombosis has reduced. You may also be given daily injections of a low-dose anticoagulant such as heparin (see p.41) until you leave hospital, although its use is not generally routine except for people who are at particular risk of thrombosis. Occasionally, the injections need to be continued at home, administered each day by a district nurse.

Leg exercises

When you come round from the anaesthetic, you can start to do some simple exercises to help the circulation of blood in your legs and to reduce the risk of deep vein thrombosis. These exercises should be done at regular intervals while you are immobile in bed, ideally for at least two minutes every hour. The physiotherapist will explain them to you.

*   Lying on your back, flex and extend your feet towards and away from your body several times. Then rotate them at the ankles in circular movements.

ANTIBIOTICS

You will probably be given an injection of antibiotic with the anaesthetic before your operation, and two more at eight-hourly intervals after it. The use of antibiotics **prophylactically** in this way is important to help reduce the risk of infection in the replaced joint. Deep infection following knee replacement is a devastating complication and usually requires removal or exchange of the prosthesis (see p.83).

EATING AND DRINKING

You are unlikely to feel like eating anything until the day after your operation and should only have sips of water for the first few post-operative hours. Drinking too much immediately after surgery can make any feeling of sickness worse. You will be able to eat normally again as soon as you want to.

DRIPS AND DRAINS

When you regain consciousness after your operation, there may be an intravenous drip in your arm to provide a specially balanced solution to replace the fluids which were lost from your body during surgery. The drip can usually be taken down after 24 to 48 hours, as soon as you are able to eat and drink normally and a blood test has shown your haemoglobin level to be normal (see p.66). It may be kept in place longer if you are likely to need a blood transfusion.

Instead of an intravenous solution, you may be given an **autologous blood transfusion** during the first 24 hours or so after your operation. A tourniquet is used during the operation itself to prevent the knee filling with blood, but once this has been removed, there is usually considerable blood loss. A process of re-infusion is therefore sometimes used – routinely in some hospitals – to collect the blood from the knee, filter it to remove any debris, and re-introduce it via a cannula inserted in an arm.

If this system of autologous blood transfusion is not used in your hospital, the excess fluid and blood will be drained away from the wound via one or more small drainage tubes. The tubes are inserted near the wound, may be held in place with a stitch, and drain into a bag or bottle. They will be removed when wound leakage reduces, usually within about 48 hours. Their removal can be uncomfortable. If you do have wound drains, you may need to have a conventional blood transfusion to replace the blood lost.

WOUND DRESSINGS AND STITCHES

There will be a protective dressing on the wound over your knee which will be checked regularly and changed as required. If your wound is still covered when you leave hospital, arrangements will be made for a district or community nurse to visit you at home to change the dressing.

Your wound may have been closed with staples, clips or stitches. Staples and clips can usually be removed after about seven days and replaced with adhesive strips to support the wound edges until healing is complete. Stitches will probably need to remain in place for about 14 days and if you have already left hospital by this time, can be removed by a district nurse at your home. A wound over the front of the knee is placed under quite substantial stress when the joint is bent, and the stitches must therefore be kept in long enough to avoid the wound bursting open before it has healed completely.

Some people are quite shocked when they see the length of their wound after knee replacement surgery. However, when you consider that the surgical incision made in the knee has to be large enough to enable the surgeon to cut away the damaged ends of the bones and insert the prosthesis, it is not surprising that it is 20 to 25 cm (8 to 10 inches) long.

TESTS AND EXAMINATIONS

For the first couple of days after your operation, you will probably have a cuff around your arm, attached to a machine which takes regular readings of your blood pressure. The cuff inflates automatically (which may be a little uncomfortable) at preset intervals – probably every quarter of an hour to begin with, then half-hourly, and then every four hours. Each blood pressure reading remains displayed until the next measurement is taken. There may also be a thermometer under your arm to take regular measurements of your body temperature in the same way. Nursing staff can thus check your blood pressure and temperature as required to monitor your condition.

Although the body temperature is often raised for a few days after surgery, a consistently raised temperature may indicate an infection, the cause of which will need to be investigated. Some people are **hypothermic** (i.e. have a low body temperature) immediately after surgery, and if necessary they can be wrapped in a foil blanket for an hour or two to bring their temperature back to normal. A high temperature post-operatively can usually be reduced by placing a fan beside the bed.

The following tests will probably be done during the first couple of post-operative days.

Blood tests

A sample of your blood may be taken the morning after your operation or after 48 hours so that its level of haemoglobin can be measured. If the haemoglobin is below normal, you may be started on a course of iron tablets. If it is significantly reduced, you may need to have a blood transfusion. Haemoglobin is important as it transports oxygen around the body which is vital to the process of wound healing (see p.16).

X-rays

An X-ray will be taken of your knee, either before you leave the operating theatre or within 24 to 48 hours post-operatively. You may have to remain in bed until this has been done. The X-ray will be kept for comparison with those taken later so that any changes can be detected.

BLADDER FUNCTION

Until you are able to get out of bed and walk to the toilet, you will be given a bedpan as required.

Urinary problems can sometimes arise in the immediate post-operative period. For example, epidurals often cause urinary retention: the bladder is unable to empty spontaneously and becomes full of urine which cannot be expelled. If this occurs, you are likely to be given a course of antibiotics to reduce the risk of infection, and a urinary catheter may be inserted through your urethra and into your bladder to drain the urine from it. The catheter will probably remain in place until you are mobile and can urinate voluntarily again.

Because epidural analgesia causes loss of sensation in the lower body, it can result in temporary incontinence. If this occurs, a urinary catheter may be inserted to drain your bladder, probably for 48 to 72 hours, and you will be given antibiotic cover.

WASHING AND DRESSING

If your wound is covered by a plastic film dressing, it may be possible for you to have showers before the stitches have been removed, although you may be advised to wait a couple of weeks to avoid the risk of infection being introduced through the wound before it has healed. Baths are best avoided for at least 10 to 12 weeks after your operation. Until you are fully mobile, you can keep clean by having regular strip washes. A nurse will help to wash your feet until you are able to bend your leg again.

There are various dressing aids available – such as long-handled shoehorns, hooked dressing sticks and stocking aids – which you may find useful, particularly if you have arthritis in other joints. The occupational therapist will explain their use to you, and you will be able to borrow any appropriate ones to use at home for a few weeks.

(a) (b)

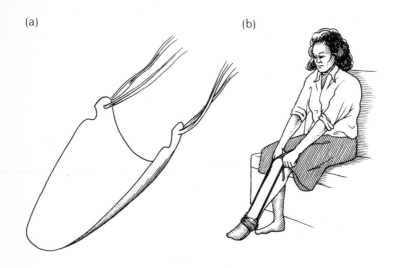

A stocking aid.

The bathrooms on the hospital ward are likely to have raised toilet seats which will make using the toilet easier, at least until you are able to bend your leg again. If you have a low-level toilet at home, the occupational therapist should be able to arrange for you to borrow a similar raised toilet seat or free-standing toilet rails to use for the first few post-operative weeks if necessary.

REHABILITATION UNITS

There are occasionally people who regain mobility slowly after knee replacement surgery, normally because they lack confidence. If medical staff think you will be unable to manage when the time comes for you to be discharged from hospital, you may be transferred to a rehabilitation unit for a few days before making the transition back home.

Rehabilitation units are staffed by nurses and normally have individual bedrooms, communal dining and sitting rooms and a kitchen where you can make drinks and snacks. Intensive efforts will be made by physiotherapists and occupational therapists to help you to strengthen your leg muscles with exercises and to regain mobility and confidence by practising walking and various everyday activities.

GOING HOME

Before you go home, the hospital staff must be satisfied that you will be able to manage. A medical social worker (see p.43) may visit you on the ward to discuss the help available through the social services, such as 'meals on wheels' or a home help. Do mention any potential problems to the medical social worker, occupational therapist or nursing staff *before* you leave hospital so that the social services can be alerted in good time if you are going to need assistance.

When you are discharged from hospital, you may be given a letter to take to your family doctor or it may be sent directly to him or her by the hospital. This discharge letter will provide all the relevant information about your operation and any follow-up treatment you require, such as the changing of a wound dressing or the removal of stitches. It should be delivered to your doctor's surgery as soon as possible.

By the time you are discharged from hospital you should have enough mobility in your knee to enable you to get in and out of a car, although you will not, of course, be able to drive. It is helpful if the person collecting you from hospital has already pushed back the passenger seat of the car to give you plenty of leg room and has made sure the floor area in front of the seat is clear of all debris, bags etc.

CHAPTER 9

Exercises and rehabilitation

Once the surgeon has replaced and/or reconstructed your knee joint, the amount of movement you regain in it depends largely on the effort you put into your rehabilitation. You will have to continue to do exercises at intervals throughout the day for the next three months at least. Surgery can cure the pain caused by a damaged or diseased knee joint, but without regular exercising maximum mobility will not return: you may have a pain-free but relatively immobile knee for the rest of your life.

It is not unusual to feel lethargic and possibly a bit depressed after any type of operation, and it may be difficult to motivate yourself to do the necessary exercises, particularly if your knee is painful. But it really is worth making the effort. Continuing to take pain-killing tablets regularly for a few weeks should control the pain and enable you to do the exercises. However, you must only do the exercises you have been told to do and, if you find them painful, you should stop immediately and ask the advice of your physiotherapist or doctor.

The knee bends at an angle of about 68 degrees during normal walking, 90 to 95 degrees when walking up and down stairs, and 95 degrees when sitting and when standing from sitting. You should be able to bend your knee by at least 80 to 90 degrees by the time you are discharged from hospital. If you cannot, additional physiotherapy may be necessary (see below). Even if you lead a relatively sedentary life and your main concern when undergoing total knee replacement was to relieve

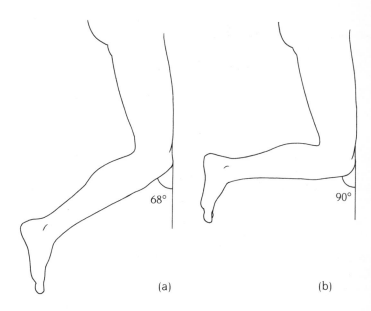

Knee flexion. (a) The angle of 68 degrees shown is the amount of flexion required during normal walking. (b) Flexion of at least 90 degrees is needed to walk up and down stairs, and this is the ideal degree of flexion aimed at before discharge from hospital.

pain which was not controlled by other forms of treatment and drugs, you will need to regain sufficient flexion in your knee to enable you to get about reasonably well and to manage your normal activities of daily living. So, whatever your situation, some exercises will be necessary.

THE PHYSIOTHERAPIST

A physiotherapist will probably visit you on the ward daily throughout your stay in hospital to help you recover mobility. In the first few days after an operation, when they are in unfamiliar surroundings and recovering from anaesthesia, many people find it difficult to concentrate, and therefore the information given to you by your physiotherapist may be repeated several times while you are in hospital.

The physiotherapist will make an assessment of your pattern of gait both before and after your operation and will draw up a programme of exercises – to do in hospital and at home – tailored to your individual needs, age and level of activity. You will be given clear instructions about the exercises you need to do. It is important that you do them properly and continue them at home, so if there is anything you do not understand, do ask the physiotherapist to explain it to you again.

If you have had knee problems for many months (or even years), you will have developed an abnormal gait and length of stride which will need to be corrected post-operatively. The height of any walking aids you use may also have to be adjusted.

Different people progress at different rates and some have particular problems or disabilities other than those related specifically to their knee problem. These factors will be taken into account by the physiotherapist in planning your rehabilitation programme, so do make sure you mention any problems which are not immediately apparent.

REGAINING MOVEMENT AND MUSCLE STRENGTH

It is important to improve the strength in the quadriceps muscle, which controls extension (straightening) of the knee and which runs down the front of it, and of the hamstring muscles, which control flexion (bending) of the knee and which run down the back of it. People who suffer from rheumatoid arthritis usually find flexing the knee easier than extending it. For those with osteoarthritis, flexion is often more difficult.

If your knee is very swollen, or you have some other problem, the programme of exercises devised for you by the physiotherapist may be adjusted. You will be shown how to do some exercises in bed after your operation, but do not start them until your physiotherapist tells you that it is safe to do so. To gain the maximum advantage, the exercises should be done for a few minutes every hour whenever you are awake. The physiotherapist will be looking for daily improvement in the range of motion of your knee joint, which should be apparent if you stick to your exercise routine as far as possible.

It is important that some strength is built up in your quadriceps before you get out of bed for the first time so that your knee does not bend abruptly when you try to walk, which could split the wound open. If, despite doing these exercises, little power develops in your leg muscles, a splint may be put on your knee while you are up until sufficient control returns. The first two exercises below are aimed specifically at strengthening the quadriceps.

By about the second post-operative day, the object of physiotherapy will be to maintain full extension of your leg and to try to regain flexion in it. Except when doing exercise 2 below, you should not rest your knee on a pillow or similar object. If the knee is held in a bent position – which may be tempting to relieve discomfort – it may eventually be unable to straighten properly: walking will then require more energy than normal and additional strain will be placed on other joints.

You will probably be able to start some exercises to strengthen the hamstring muscles (exercise 4 below) on the second post-operative day.

All the following exercises should be done hourly if possible, *unless you are told otherwise*.

Exercise 1
Lie or sit on the bed with your legs straight. Tighten the muscles in your thigh so that the back of the knee presses onto the bed. Hold them tight for 5 seconds. Repeat ten times.

Exercise 2
Put a rolled-up blanket under your operated knee and, keeping your thigh on the blanket, try to lift your heel as high as you can. Hold it up for 2 seconds and then slowly lower it again. Start by doing this exercise five times, gradually increasing the number you can do.

Exercise 3
Keeping your thigh muscles clenched and your leg straight, practise raising the whole of your leg off the bed. You will probably not be told to do this exercise if your knee is very painful.

Exercise 4
Place a sliding board under your foot, and slide your heel up it, bending your knee towards you as far as it will go. Then lower your leg by sliding your heel back down the board. Repeat this exercise ten times.

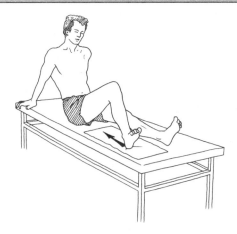

Exercise 4.

By about day four after your operation, you may be able to add some more exercises to your routine, but do not do so until your physiotherapist says you can.

Exercise 5
Sit on the edge of your bed with your back straight. Cross your legs at the ankles, with your **un**operated leg over your operated one. Use the **un**operated leg to push the operated one gently back until you feel the muscles stretching. Hold it there for 10 seconds and then relax. Repeat this exercise five times to help improve flexion in your knee joint.

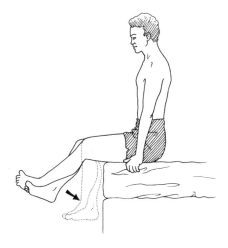

Exercise 5.

Exercise 6
Lie on the bed with your shoulders raised and resting on your elbows. Place a folded pillow between your knees and press them together. Hold this position for 10 seconds and then relax. Repeat this exercise three times to help improve your muscle strength.

Exercise 7
Stand with your hands holding on to something solid or resting against a wall and place your operated leg in front of your **un**operated leg. Lunge forwards, bending your operated leg as much as possible. Hold this position for 5 seconds and then relax. Repeat five times. This exercise helps to improve the movement in your knee but should *not* be done if it is swollen or bruised or if you have any problem with the wound.

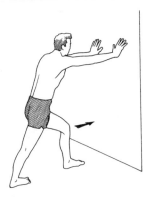

Exercise 7.

GETTING OUT OF BED

One or two physiotherapists will help you to get out of bed for the first time, probably on the second day after your operation. Your legs are likely to seem weak to begin with and you may feel dizzy or faint when you first try to get up. Do say immediately if this is the case as it is much easier and safer to put you back on the bed before you actually faint. It is important not to attempt to get out of bed without the assistance of a physiotherapist or nurse for the first few times at least. If you are using patient-controlled analgesia (see p.55) or have an epidural for pain relief, getting you up may be delayed until it has been removed.

As you extend your leg over the side of the bed, a physiotherapist may support your calf to prevent the knee bending suddenly. Once you are up, and as long as you do not feel faint, the physiotherapist(s) will help you to walk a short distance using a walking frame.

In some hospitals, it is routine practice for people to wear leg braces for the first few post-operative days whenever they are out of bed to help support the knee.

ADDITIONAL PHYSIOTHERAPY

There are various methods of physiotherapy to help strengthen the leg muscles and improve mobility of the knee joint after knee replacement surgery. Some are used routinely in some hospitals, and some are brought into action when problems arise.

Continuous passive motion

Continuous passive motion machines move the leg up and

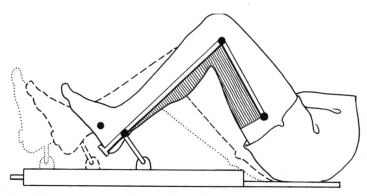

A continuous passive motion machine. The machine bends the knee without the need for active movement of the muscles. It is sometimes used after surgery to assist flexion.

down continuously while it rests on a frame-like structure of adjustable length. The machine can aid wound healing but cannot replace the need for active movement or the exercises described above.

Where continuous passive motion machines are not used routinely, they may be available for people who had a poor range of movement of the knee before their operation and for those whose post-operative progress is slow.

Cryotherapy

Your knee may be quite swollen for four weeks or more after your operation, but the exercises you do should help reduce the swelling. If necessary, cryotherapy can be used, both in hospital and at home.

Cryotherapy is simply the application of ice to reduce swelling, inflammation or bruising. The ice should never come in direct contact with the skin as it could cause 'ice burns'. It should therefore always be wrapped in a damp towel and it is a good idea also to put a little oil or oily lotion on the skin first to protect it. When you are at home you can hold broken ice cubes or a pack of frozen peas wrapped in a damp tea towel on your knee while you sit with your leg raised. (It is best to use small pieces of ice or small frozen vegetables to avoid 'burning' the skin.) Any packs of frozen vegetables used in this way should be clearly marked to ensure that they are not eaten after having been defrosted and refrozen.

Flowtron

A flowtron is a giant, inflatable splint which was originally developed to treat **oedema** – swelling caused by the collection of fluid in part of the body. It can also be zipped up around the leg to stretch it, and is sometimes used pre-operatively for six to eight hours a day. Once the wound has healed sufficiently not to burst open when pressure is applied – usually about six days or more after surgery – it may also be used post-operatively. The flowtron may be left in place for about two hours a day, or is sometimes used overnight.

Hydrotherapy

In hospitals with a hydrotherapy pool, gentle exercise in water may be routine or it may be used when progress is slow, from day four or five after surgery. If you are having hydrotherapy, your wound will be protected by a waterproof dressing.

SURGICAL MANIPULATION

Sometimes, surgical manipulation is undertaken under anaesthesia to help improve the range of motion of the knee. The surgeon bends the knee to break down **adhesions** which have formed and which are preventing it moving through its normal range of motion. Most people are then put on a continuous passive motion machine in the recovery room and remain on it for about 24 hours, or until they can move their knee spontaneously. Surgical manipulation usually involves at least a couple of days in hospital and is sometimes followed by hydrotherapy or some other physiotherapy procedure.

Surgical manipulation is best done about four to six weeks after surgery before too much scar tissue has built up in the knee. Some people who have failed to regain much flexion in the knee and who are still in hospital four or five weeks after their operation may undergo manipulation under anaesthesia before they are discharged. For others, it may be considered at their first follow-up appointment, some six weeks or so after surgery, if little further progress has been made since they were discharged.

CHAPTER 10

After your operation: at home

By the time you leave hospital, you should be reasonably mobile and able to do most things for yourself at home. You will be given any necessary advice, including how and when to use your walking aids. You will probably have progressed from walking with a walking frame to using two sticks. It may be several weeks before you can manage with only one walking stick, which should be held in the hand opposite your operated leg.

Apart from taking sensible precautions, particularly during the first three months or so after your operation, there will be few long-term restrictions on what you are able to do. You should not kneel on your operated leg for at least six months as there is little flesh over the knee cap and putting pressure on it in this way could re-open the wound and will certainly be uncomfortable. If you do have to kneel briefly for any reason, do so on a cushion or some sort of padding. You should avoid all heavy manual labour such as digging etc. until your consultant tells you it is safe to do it. You will therefore have to have several weeks off work if your job entails this sort of activity.

DAILY ACTIVITIES

To gain any real benefit from your operation, you will have to continue to do your exercises regularly for about three months, after which you can increase the natural function of your leg while gradually decreasing the time you spend exercising. However, if your knee begins to stiffen at any time, you should use it less and exercise it more. In some cases, exercises have to be continued in the long term to retain movement in the knee joint. If you have any specific mobility problems, you may be given hydrotherapy or special exercises to do for some time after your operation or you may continue to see a physiotherapist at regular out-patient appointments to deal with a particular difficulty.

It is important that you keep reasonably active, without over-doing it. You will need someone to do your shopping and heavy housework for a couple of weeks at least. During the first few post-operative weeks, you should avoid standing for long periods and do jobs such as ironing or preparing meals while sitting down. The effort and care you put into your rehabilitation programme will help you make good and steady progress.

* *Walking*. Walking is very good exercise – in moderation – but you should avoid walking on uneven or slippery surfaces. If walking or standing causes your knee to swell, restart the exercises instead.

* *Sitting*. Avoid sitting in the same position for long periods of time as doing so may cause your knee to stiffen. If you do sit for any length of time, alternate between resting your leg on a stool and placing your foot on the floor.

* *Going up and down stairs*. Your physiotherapist will have prac-tised going up and down stairs with you before you left hos-pital if this was thought necessary. When going up stairs, place your **un**operated leg on each stair first, then your oper-ated leg and then your walking stick. When going down stairs, the sequence is walking stick first, then your operated leg and then your **un**operated leg. You may be able to man-age to go up and down stairs normally after about six weeks.

* *Washing and dressing*. You can have showers or baths once your stitches have been removed or if your wound is

covered with a waterproof dressing. Showers are preferable until the wound has healed as they present less risk of infection than baths.

Until you have regained good flexion in your knee joint, or if you have arthritis in other joints, you may find it difficult to bend your leg to cut your toenails, put on your shoes and socks etc. Therefore, if necessary, you will be given any useful dressing aids before you leave hospital (see p.67).

* *Driving*. You may be able to resume driving after your first follow-up appointment – at six to eight weeks post-operatively – but you should not drive until your consultant says it is safe to do so. Even if you have regained sufficient movement in your knee joint, your reflexes may not be back to normal for several weeks. Driving should be avoided for three or four months following revision surgery.

The terms of your insurance policy may require you to let your insurance company know that you have had knee replacement surgery before you start driving again. This is a stipulation with some types of insurance, and failing to comply with it could mean that you are not covered should you have an accident, possibly even several months after your operation. It is therefore worth checking with your insurance company – and asking for their answer in writing – even if you think this rule does not apply in your case.

* *Sport*. Swimming is a good form of exercise after a knee replacement operation, unless you are advised against it for some reason. You may be able to return to doing gentle sporting activities by about six to eight weeks after your operation, but must be able to walk without walking aids before you do so. If your knee swells or becomes painful, stop all sports and start to do your exercises again. It is best to ask your consultant's advice before resuming a sport which involves standing. *Vigorous sports are never appropriate*

after knee replacement surgery and therefore you will be unable to play squash, badminton or any other sport which places a repetitive impact load on the joint, although you should be able to play golf.

FOLLOW-UP APPOINTMENTS

You will probably have an out-patient appointment about six to eight weeks after your operation so that your knee can be examined and an X-ray taken of it. Another appointment will probably be made for about six months after surgery, during which further X-rays will be taken and you will be assessed by the surgeon and a physiotherapist. By this time you should have regained enough mobility and muscle strength to allow you to resume your normal daily activities.

During the weeks following your knee replacement operation, do make a note of any questions you wish to ask and take it with you to your follow-up appointment.

The risk of infection The large components of a replaced knee lie immediately beneath the skin and are not protected by soft tissues. The joint is therefore vulnerable to infection, either introduced through the wound before it has healed or via infective organisms which have travelled in the blood from elsewhere in the body. Infection is a very serious complication when it occurs following joint replacement. If it spreads to the knee, the replaced joint may have to be removed and it is not always possible for new prostheses to be inserted. It is therefore essential that you contact your doctor or the hospital immediately should you have any problems with the wound, such as discharge or breakdown, or if you develop any type of infection – a chest infection, ear infection, infected cut etc. – however minor it may seem to you. You will need to have antibiotic cover to prevent it spreading. Always err on the side of caution.

CHAPTER 11

Possible post-operative complications

There are some general complications which can occur after any type of operation, and some which are specifically related to knee replacement surgery. Most complications are minor, but occasionally more serious ones arise. Apart from those which may develop within hours or days of surgery, there are others which may not become apparent for months, or even years. It is therefore important to be aware of what could go wrong and to seek medical attention if you are at all concerned.

GENERAL COMPLICATIONS

The general complications described here can occur in some form after any operation and, where necessary, precautions will be taken to reduce their risk.

Chest infection

Chest infection is possible following general anaesthesia, and is particularly common in smokers. Deep breathing is important post-operatively to keep the lungs clear and, if necessary, a physiotherapist will visit you on the ward to advise you about appropriate exercises.

Pyrexia

Pyrexia is fever. It is quite normal for it to develop in the first 24 to 72 hours after surgery, but if it persists its cause will have to be investigated. Amongst other causes, pyrexia can be due to a chest or wound infection or to deep vein thrombosis (see below).

Thrombosis and embolism

Deep vein thrombosis occurs when a blood clot forms in one of the deep veins of the body – usually in the calf veins of the legs. Its potential danger is associated with the risk of the blood clot breaking away and lodging, for example, in the lungs, causing a pulmonary embolism (see p.39).

It has been estimated, in both the UK and the USA, that approximately 50 per cent of people undergoing surgery to the lower extremities develop deep vein thrombosis. This relatively high incidence is partly due to the fact that surgery involving bone releases a substance called **thromboplastin** which plays a role in the natural process of the formation of blood clots. Surgery can also cause distension of the valve cusps which control the flow of blood through the blood vessels, thus leading to the pooling of blood (known as **stasis**) within the veins of the leg.

Precautions such as the wearing of anti-embolism stockings (see p.40), a course of low-dose heparin or warfarin injections to thin the blood and help prevent clotting (see p.41), exercises and, importantly, becoming mobile as soon as possible after your operation should help to prevent thrombosis.

Thrombosis in the *calf* rarely leads to pulmonary embolism (which is associated more commonly with thrombosis in the *thigh*), but it is important to be aware of its signs and symptoms and to seek medical attention immediately. A blood clot may be symptomless, possibly developing 48 hours or more after surgery, or it may give rise to local tenderness, swelling, fever and pain. Treatment will be necessary to avoid further complications; pulmonary embolism is more difficult to treat. Treatment of a thrombus in the calf usually involves bed rest and elevation of the affected leg, with or without the use of intravenous heparin or warfarin. Deep vein thrombosis in the thigh will need to be very carefully monitored in hospital and higher-dose heparin or warfarin injections will sometimes have to be continued for three months or longer.

Pain

For some people, the gradual easing of immediate post-operative pain does not occur. For most of them, the pain associated with surgery and with exercises to stretch the muscles around the knee will cease once the operative area heals and stabilises and a good range of motion has been achieved. It is particularly important that any pain is well controlled after a knee replacement operation so that the exercises necessary to regain function in the joint can be done. There are various methods of pain relief available, including the regular use of analgesic tablets and physiotherapy.

Despite analgesia, a small percentage of people experience persistent pain for no obvious reason and it may be that some of them, at least, have a low pain threshold. If pain continues, or increases, investigations may need to be done to rule out the presence of a collection of blood (known as a haematoma, see p.90), infection or any other physical cause.

Superficial wound infection

Infection sometimes occurs in the wound following any operation. Primary wound healing is important and if your wound continues to ooze a bloody discharge, you may be started on a course of antibiotics and kept in hospital until it has completely healed. Occasionally, germs collect around the stitches, some of which may have to be removed to allow an infected discharge to escape. A superficial wound infection may rapidly progress to a deep infection of the knee (see below) because the prosthesis lies just beneath the skin. Any problems with the wound must therefore be brought to the attention of a nurse or doctor.

It is possible for an infection to arise even weeks or months after surgery if foreign bodies such as suture material have been left within the wound. Infection can also develop in a wound as a result of spread of infective organisms from elsewhere in the body, when it is known as **metastatic infection**.

You should seek medical attention if you have the following signs: pain, swelling, heat and redness around the wound, possibly with leakage of pus or infected fluid, and a high body temperature.

Deep infection

Infection is always a risk when materials are implanted into the body. Operating theatres in which knee replacement surgery takes place are therefore fitted with special ventilation systems to clean the air. In some centres, operating staff also wear body suits, similar in appearance to space suits. Before the first incision is made during the operation, the operation site is always cleaned with an antiseptic solution and the patient's body is covered with sterile drapes.

Antibiotics are normally given for 24 hours before and after surgery, and sometimes for longer. For people at high risk (and often routinely), the cement used to fix an implant may be impregnated with antibiotic which leaches out over the following weeks to provide some additional protection against the multiplication of bacteria in the immediate area.

Sepsis is infection caused by pus-producing organisms. Once present, it is difficult to cure. Deep sepsis is catastrophic and usually leads to joint failure, with the need to remove the replaced knee joint to control the infection. Depending on the severity of the infection and the organisms involved, a new knee joint may either be inserted at the time of removal of the old one or 6 to 12 weeks later. However, replacing the prosthesis is not always successful and sepsis may cause long-term disability.

Despite the precautions taken, the main cause of sepsis is contamination of the wound during surgery, either with airborne bacteria or with bacteria transferred from the patient's skin. It may also occur after surgery if bacteria are transferred to the operation site via the blood or lymph from a urinary tract infection, skin break or abscess etc. Therefore, the skin over the operating site is always examined carefully before surgery and if there are any skin breaks or abrasions, the operation may be postponed until they have healed. Surgery may also be postponed if, when your mouth is examined pre-operatively, you are found to require dental repairs (see p.17). A sample of your urine will be analysed before your operation to detect the presence of any urinary tract infection (see p.16). The risk of postoperative sepsis may also be increased if there is a delay in wound healing.

Although the incidence of sepsis immediately after knee surgery is declining, due to the precautionary measures described, it does still occur, even a year or more after surgery and sometimes because an infection has remained latent since a previous operation or injury.

People at increased risk of sepsis include those with autoimmune diseases, rheumatoid arthritis, systemic lupus erythematosus or diabetes, as well as those who are corticosteroid dependent. Its incidence doubles following revision surgery.

Swelling

Swelling and warmth of the knee are quite common for some time after surgery. Although they are normal reactions to overuse of the knee joint, they should be reported to your doctor or consultant for investigation if accompanied by an increase in pain and a limited range of motion as they could be due to a low-level infection which will have to be treated with antibiotics.

It is not uncommon for swelling to develop in the calf, ankle or foot after knee replacement surgery. Although, again, this is rarely a cause for concern, it may need to be investigated as it could be an early sign of a deep vein thrombosis (see p.85).

Nerve damage

The small nerves supplying the skin over the operation site are usually damaged when an incision is made during surgery, occasionally causing a small area around the wound to remain permanently numb. Although the size of the area of numbness will decrease with time, the sensation may never return completely.

Neuroma

Very rarely, small, painful, tender areas form in part of the scar, which may be due to a swelling of the cut nerve ends known as a neuroma. Nerve damage may lead to pain in the wound which will be relieved temporarily by the injection of local anaesthetic. Continued pain may respond to steroid injection. Only rarely is surgery needed to remove a painful nodule.

Nerve palsy

The nerve damage which can occur during an operation can cause loss of sensation, and possibly power, which may last for days or months but which will eventually recover to a greater or lesser extent as the nerves regenerate. However, depending on the damage to the nerves, they may never fully repair themselves and loss of function of the affected part – known as nerve palsy – can develop. Nerve palsy is more common in women (for reasons which are not fully understood) and following revision surgery. The nerve most commonly damaged after total knee replacement is that which supplies the muscles involved in lifting the foot at the ankle.

Bleeding and bruising

There is often a certain amount of oozing of blood or fluid from the wound, but this is unlikely to be heavy. If it continues, and particularly if leakage occurs through the wound dressing and soils your clothes, medical advice should be sought. On rare occasions, a second operation is required to tie off or cauterise a bleeding blood vessel which was overlooked or which has started to bleed again post-operatively.

Occasionally, blood which does not escape through the edges of the wound may give rise to severe bruising, possibly several days after surgery. Although the sight of the bruise may be distressing, treatment is only seldom required to release the blood which has accumulated under the skin.

Haematoma

In rare cases, a haematoma may develop. A haematoma is a swelling which is full of blood and is caused by a blood vessel either continuing to bleed or re-opening after surgery, or by a collection of blood oozing into a space created during surgery. It can sometimes result from a disturbance of the normal blood-clotting mechanisms of the body, for example caused by anti-coagulants such as heparin. There are also inherited bleeding disorders, such as haemophilia, which cause a similar disturbance of the blood-clotting mechanisms, but these conditions will be taken into account before any operation is considered.

The formation of a haematoma is accompanied by pain, the development of a hard swelling, and possibly a reddish purple discoloration of the skin. Bruising may appear around the wound or at some distance from it over the next few days. A raised body temperature may result from the haematoma itself or from infection in the wound (see above).

If you think a haematoma is forming once you have left hospital, you should contact your family doctor or consultant for advice. The blood is likely to be reabsorbed spontaneously within three or four weeks without the need for any treatment, but if heavy bleeding continues, with increased pain and swelling, you may need surgery to close off the blood vessel which is causing it. Your doctor may also wish to do specialised blood tests to check that your blood-clotting factors are normal.

COMPLICATIONS OF KNEE REPLACEMENT SURGERY

Apart from the general complications of surgery described above, the following are specifically related to knee replacement surgery. In most cases, the risk is increased after revision surgery.

Patella dislocation

Dislocation of the knee cap can occur following knee replacement surgery, and is almost always lateral. **Subluxation** (incomplete dislocation) is also possible, although less common, and may cause difficulty bending the leg. Some form of soft tissue release and re-alignment is usually required in persistent cases.

Instability of the knee joint

Occasionally, the knee can be felt or seen to slip when held in various positions. Wearing a brace around the knee and doing exercises to strengthen the quadriceps and hamstring muscles are usually enough to cure this instability. Very rarely, the problem is sufficiently severe to lead to subluxation or functional problems, in which case surgery may be required to replace the prostheses partially or completely and so restore stability to the joint.

Joint noise

Although some form of noise from the knee joint is common following total knee replacement, it is only rarely accompanied by pain and does not usually require any treatment. The clicks and other sounds which may be heard occur as the prostheses move in relation to each other and in most cases subside with time.

Flexion contracture

A pre-existing deformity or weak quadriceps muscle may interfere with the ability to straighten the knee fully after surgery. If this problem is not dealt with promptly, the bend in the knee becomes fixed – a so-called flexion contracture.

Heterotopic bone formation

Heterotopic bone formation is the development of bone in an area of the body in which it is not normally produced. It may occur within the soft tissues around the knee, or it may protrude in spurs from the end of the femur or tibia. When severe, it may limit the degree of flexion of the knee, requiring manipulation or surgical removal. Surgery will usually be delayed for six months or more to allow the bone to mature fully. However, it is a very rare complication following knee replacement surgery.

Aseptic loosening

In the past, it was not unusual for a component of a replaced knee joint to fail, but this risk has been much reduced by the use of stronger modern alloys and improved design. However, the plastic bearing surface may still wear significantly over 10 to 15 years.

Aseptic loosening (i.e. loosening of the components of a replaced knee caused by something other than infection) may be the result of a less-than-perfect surgical technique, poor quality or quantity of the bone to which the prosthesis has been attached, excessive body weight, or inappropriate or excessive activity, all of which may lead to absorption and breakdown of the bone (osteolysis).

Failure may occur between the cement or porous coating and the bone, or between the prosthesis and the cement. Where possible, aseptic loosening is treated by revising the knee replacement.

Foreign body reaction

A problem with plastic components is that they may wear, producing debris which can cause a foreign body reaction. Degradation of cement can also lead to resorption of the bone stock and thus component loosening (see above). The debris may lead to osteolysis in the tibia or femur which is usually associated with pain and loosening of the implant.

Fracture

Very rarely, a knee replacement operation may fail due to fracture of the femur or tibia. Sometimes loosening of an implant, associated with osteolysis (see above), weakens the bone stock and may predispose to fracture. Fractures may also result from post-operative injury or trauma, bone disorders or osteoporosis (see p.9). Osteoporotic bone may fracture at the junction between the stiff implant and the soft bone, particularly in the lower part of the femur. Fracture is more common after revision surgery and may also occur *during* surgery if the operation is difficult to perform or the bone is weakened for any reason.

CHAPTER 12

Revision surgery

Sometimes knee replacements fail, possibly (but not commonly) as a result of infection or some other complication, or because the components have worn with the passage of time. If failure occurs, revision surgery will be necessary to remove the primary knee replacement and insert new components. Although it is possible to repeat revision surgery – in theory, at least, as many times as necessary – the results do tend to become progressively less good. The amount of scar tissue produced after any type of surgery increases with each successive operation. Following even a first revision operation, the muscles of the leg may not work as well as they did after the primary knee replacement, and occasional aches in the legs are relatively common. In many respects, the details of the preparation for and recovery from revision surgery are similar to those of primary knee replacement, but some aspects of the two types of operation do differ and the effort required for successful rehabilitation will certainly be greater.

BEFORE THE OPERATION

The pre-operative tests done prior to revision surgery are basically the same as those described in Chapter 2. Before revision surgery is undertaken, it is very important that any existing infection is detected and treated. Infection present in the primary replaced knee could recur in the revised knee, possibly causing the components to loosen. Therefore, you are likely to have blood tests, isotope scans (see p.17) and **aspiration** to detect infective organisms in your knee joint or elsewhere in your body. Aspiration may be done under a local or general anaesthetic and involves the insertion of a needle into the knee to remove a sample of fluid from it, which is then examined for the presence of bacteria.

THE OPERATION

The operation involves essentially the same approach as for primary knee replacement. However, it is often more difficult to dislocate the patella laterally because of the presence of extensive scar tissue. It is necessary to do a fairly extensive dissection to break down both the scar tissue and the adhesions so that the joint can be mobilised and access can be obtained to all parts of the knee to remove the components and replace them.

Loss of bone sometimes requires bone grafting, with or without fixation with screws. Alternatively, lost bone can be replaced by special wedges which are attached to the artificial components themselves. Many knee systems used in primary knee replacement are designed to accept special knee revision components.

Where the ligaments around the knee are damaged or stretched, the prostheses may have to be constrained (like a hinge) to provide stability to the knee. Although this is sometimes necessary, it is undesirable as it creates an increased strain at the fixation point which may lead to loosening of the prostheses. Where it is not necessary, the prostheses are cemented in place in the same way as for primary knee replacement and the wound is closed in a routine manner (see p.60).

AFTER THE OPERATION

The post-operative care and rehabilitation following revision surgery are similar to those after a primary operation, although you may be in hospital for a little longer. Because there is likely to be more scar tissue, you will have to work harder to regain movement after a revision operation and it is very important that you do the necessary exercises regularly. Even so, you may never achieve as much movement in the knee joint as you had after your primary operation.

You may need to use crutches for longer after revision surgery and may have to wear a knee brace to hold your new joint in position while the tissues heal.

CHAPTER 13

Private care

In countries such as Britain where there is a state health service, there are various reasons why people choose to have their operations done privately. They may have private health insurance, or be covered by a private health scheme run by the company for which they work, or they may be able to pay for private care themselves. Because the NHS waiting lists for knee replacement surgery are often quite long, and because people waiting to have this operation are usually suffering significant pain and disability, quite a substantial number are done privately. Many people who are able to choose prefer the privacy of a private hospital and to be able to enter hospital at a convenient time. As private hospitals rarely deal with accidents and emergency treatment (the operations carried out in them normally being planned at least a day or two in advance), they do not have the bustle of NHS hospitals.

If you have an operation in an NHS hospital, you may not see the consultant at all, but may be examined, treated and operated on by other doctors in the consultant's firm. At a private hospital, you will receive personal care from the consultant throughout your stay and your operation will be performed by him or her. The facilities at a private hospital are likely to be similar to those of a good hotel, and will certainly include a private bathroom.

Whatever your situation, you will not find that the *standard* of medical care you receive in a private hospital is any different from that available on the National Health Service.

The information given in other chapters in this book is equally relevant whichever system you choose. This chapter explains the practicalities of obtaining private health care and deals with the differences between the two systems.

It is possible, even if you are already on an NHS waiting list, to tell your family doctor or consultant at any time that you would like to change to private care. If the consultant you have already seen under the NHS does not have a private practice, you can ask to be put in touch with one who *can* see you privately.

PRIVATE HEALTH INSURANCE

If you work for a company which has a private health insurance scheme, your Company Secretary will be able to give you details, and should be able to tell you if the company insurance covers you for your operation.

If you have your own private health insurance, someone at the insurance company will be able to tell you exactly what is covered by your particular policy if this is not clear from the literature you already have. It is always worth checking anyway, and asking for *written* confirmation. Do not be afraid to keep asking questions until you are certain you know exactly which costs you will be responsible for paying yourself. For example, does your insurance cover all follow-up appointments?

There are different levels of health insurance, and you need to make sure you know which costs are included. Some policies have an annual maximum pay-out, so if you have had any out-patient investigations during the year, you should make sure you have not already reached your limit. Most private hospitals have an administration officer who will check your policy for you if you are in any doubt and will try to sort out any problems and queries you have. But do read your policy carefully, and any information sent to you by the hospital, as unexpected charges, such as consultants' fees which may not be covered, could add up to quite a lot of money. Some insurance policies have a ceiling cost for consultants' fees and, if the fees quoted by your consultant exceed this limit, you will have to pay the extra yourself.

With some types of private health insurance, you will need to ask your family doctor to fill in a form stating that your operation is necessary and cannot be done in an NHS hospital within a certain time period due to long waiting lists. You will have to pay your doctor for this service, which will cost a few pounds. This money is not redeemable from your insurers.

After you are discharged from hospital, you may receive accounts from the surgeon and anaesthetist. You should either send these to the hospital, for forwarding to your insurance company with their own account, or direct to your insurer, making sure you quote your policy number and the date and place of your operation in case they have not yet received the hospital account and do not have any record of your operation. Always take, and keep, a copy of all accounts and completed claim forms.

FIXED PRICE CARE

If you think you may be able to pay to have your operation done privately, the Bookings Manager at a private hospital can give you an idea of the cost involved. Some private hospitals run a service known as Fixed Price Care: a price can be quoted to you before you enter hospital which covers your operation and a variety of other hospitalisation costs. You should always ask to have the quotation in writing *before* you enter hospital, with a written note of everything it includes. At some hospitals, the fixed price will only include hospital-related costs such as accommodation, nursing, meals, drugs, dressings, operating theatre fees, X-rays etc.; at others the consultants' fees are also included. Once you have a written quotation, you should not have to worry about any hidden costs or increased costs due to any medical complications which make it necessary for you to have to stay in hospital longer than expected, usually up to a maximum of 28 days. You should ask your consultant whether his or her quoted fees (and those of the anaesthetist) would cover this eventuality.

At some hospitals, the quoted price will also include your treatment should you have to be re-admitted due to a complication related to your original operation and arising within a limited period of time after your discharge. However, if you develop some problem while in hospital which is unrelated to your original knee condition, the price you have been quoted will not cover treatment to deal with this.

The only extra charges you will have to pay to the hospital will probably include those for telephone calls, any alcohol if you have this with your meals, food provided for your visitors, personal laundry done by the hospital and any similar items such as you would have to pay for in a hotel. It is usually possible for a visitor to eat meals with you in your room, and for tea and snacks to be ordered for visitors during the day. (You will also have to pay these extra charges before you leave the hospital if you are being treated under private health insurance.)

It is important therefore that you ask in advance for *written confirmation* of the price you will have to pay for your stay in hospital and precisely what is included in the quotation. If the hospital does not have a Fixed Price Care or similar system, make sure that all possible costs are listed.

ARRANGING THE OPERATION

As for treatment under the NHS, you will have to be referred to see a consultant privately by your family doctor. Most doctors have contacts with particular consultants (and private hospitals) to whom they tend to refer patients, and private consultant surgeons (and anaesthetists) almost always have an NHS practice as well. If there is a private hospital you particularly want to go to, or a consultant you have some reason to prefer, you can ask your family doctor to make an appointment for you.

After your visit to your doctor, you are unlikely to have to wait longer than a week or two before you see the consultant at an out-patient appointment. Your appointment may be at the private hospital where your operation is to be carried out, at an NHS hospital which has private wards, or at the consultant's private consulting rooms. Once the decision has been made to go ahead with surgery, you will probably be able to enter hospital within a few weeks at most.

You will receive confirmation of the date of your operation from the Bookings Manager of the hospital you are to attend. You may also be sent leaflets and any further relevant details about your admission. Do read these carefully, as knowing how a particular hospital organises things will help you to be prepared when you arrive for your operation. You will also be sent a **pre-admission form** to fill in and take with you when you are admitted.

If your operation is being paid for by insurance, you will be asked to take a completed insurance form with you when you are admitted to hospital. You should have been given some of these forms when you first took out your policy, but your insurance company will be able to supply the correct one if you have any problems. If you are covered by company insurance, the form will probably be filled in and given to you by your Company Secretary.

ADMISSION AND DISCHARGE

When you arrive at the hospital, the receptionist will contact the admissions department, and a ward receptionist will come to collect you. If you are paying for your treatment yourself, you will probably be asked to pay your bill in advance at this stage if you have not already done so. Otherwise, you will be asked for your completed insurance form. The ward receptionist will take you to your room, which will probably be a single or double room with a private bathroom, a television, and a telephone by your bed. The ward receptionist will explain hospital procedures to you, and will leave you to settle in.

A member of the nursing staff will then come to make a note of your medical details, in much the same way as described in Chapter 5. The main difference you are likely to notice if you have been treated in an NHS hospital before, is that this time there is much less waiting for all the routine hospital procedures to be dealt with. The nurse to patient ratio is usually higher in private hospitals and so someone should be available to deal with the pre-operative procedures quite quickly.

Your consultant will take charge of your medical care throughout your stay, will visit you before the operation, perform the operation (with the assistance of the anaesthetist and the operating staff), and visit you again when you are back in your own room. Trainees – whether doctors, nurses or paramedical staff – do not work in private hospitals. The consultants are responsible for their own patients and supervise their care themselves. Most private hospitals now have resident medical officers – fully qualified, registered doctors who are available 24 hours a day to deal with any emergencies which may arise.

When the time for your operation approaches a porter and nurse will take you from your room to the anaesthetic room. In many private hospitals, you will not be moved from your bed onto a trolley until you have been anaesthetised; the bed itself will be wheeled from your room. Similarly, you will be transferred back from the trolley to your own bed in the recovery room while you are still asleep. You therefore go to sleep and wake up in your own hospital bed.

Your operation will be performed in the same way as described in Chapter 7. When you are fully awake, you will be taken back to your room to rest.

When you are ready to be discharged from hospital, the ward receptionist will ask you to pay any outstanding charges not covered by the hospitalisation charge, and you will be given any medical items you may need from the hospital pharmacy.

Questions and answers

The answers to most of these questions can be found elsewhere in the book. However, this section may help you to compile your own list to ask your family doctor or consultant. It is useful to write down questions as they occur to you, and to take your list with you to your doctor's appointment. Most people find it difficult to remember the things they want to ask when they are trying to take in information being given to them by their doctor.

The answers given here are general and specific information may differ slightly, according to the normal practice of particular surgeons and hospitals.

Always ask your family doctor, the hospital doctor who is in charge of your care, or a nurse whenever you do not understand something. No question is too trivial, particularly if it concerns something that is worrying you.

1. How long will I be in hospital following my knee replacement operation and will I be able to manage alone at home by the time I am discharged?

The length of time you are in hospital will depend in part on the progress you make and on the effort you put into your post-operative exercises. The average stay is about ten days. Before you are discharged, hospital staff will want to be sure that you have regained enough mobility in your knee to enable you to get about, go up and down stairs etc. By the time you leave hospital you should be able to do most things for yourself, but you will have to use walking sticks for several weeks, and will need someone to do your shopping and heavy housework for at least a couple of weeks. If necessary, the social services can provide assistance until you can manage alone, for example a home help and/or 'meals on wheels'. If you live alone or feel you may need some help when you are discharged from hospital, do mention it at your pre-operative assessment appointment or when you are first admitted to hospital so that the necessary arrangements can be made in good time.

2. I am on a waiting list to have knee replacement surgery but am very anxious about the prospect of being given a general anaesthetic. Is there an alternative and, if so, how can I make sure I receive it?

There *are* alternatives to general anaesthesia but your anaesthetist will decide which type of anaesthetic is most appropriate for you. Do discuss your fears with the anaesthetist at your pre-operative assessment appointment or when you are admitted to hospital for your operation as it may be possible to take your preferences into account.

General anaesthesia has improved enormously in recent years and the associated risks are now small. Your anaesthetist will be able to explain the procedures and discuss the possible complications with you. However, regional anaesthetic – either spinal or epidural – in combination with a sedative is sometimes used for knee replacement surgery and it may be possible for this type of anaesthesia to be considered for you instead.

3. I am on a waiting list to have knee replacement surgery, but have been told it may be some months before my operation can be done. How long would I have to wait to have the operation done privately and is it too late to find out about this option?

Even though you are already on an NHS waiting list for surgery, you are quite entitled to ask your family doctor for a referral to a private consultant. You will have to pay your doctor a small fee for this service.

The consultant whose NHS list you are already on may also

have a private practice, but if not your doctor can arrange for an appointment to be made for you to see a consultant who does practise privately. You will probably only have to wait a week or two for your appointment, and then not more than a few weeks at most for your operation.

Do ask the consultant for a note of what his or her fees, and those of the anaesthetist, are likely to be. You should also contact the private hospital where your operation would take place and ask for a *written* quote of the costs involved. A knee replacement operation is likely to amount to several thousand pounds.

You can remain on the NHS waiting list while you make your decision, but do let your doctor know once you decide what to do.

4. I *have had to give up playing rugby because of problems with my knee. If I have knee replacement surgery, will I be able to play sports again after it?*

Although you may regain a very good range of movement in your knee after surgery, *any* vigorous sporting activity will be inappropriate and would at the very least shorten the expected lifespan of the replaced joint. Revision surgery would probably be possible when the components fail, but would be likely to give less satisfactory results and to cause further damage to your bones and soft tissues. Knee replacement surgery is undertaken to deal with pain and disability, but never to enable people to participate in vigorous sports.

5. I *had arranged for my father to stay with me for a couple of weeks after a knee replacement operation he is due to have. However, because of unexpected work commitments, this is now unlikely to be possible. I do not want to ask for his operation to be postponed as I understand it might mean him having to wait several more months. On the other hand, I really don't think he would be able to manage alone when he is discharged from hospital. What should I do?*

Your father should mention the change of plan at his pre-operative assessment appointment. If he has already attended a pre-operative clinic, you or he could ring the hospital ward and ask whether arrangements could be made to provide assistance for him during the first couple of weeks or so after he is discharged. The social services can usually arrange support for people in their own homes, and hospitals have medical social workers on their staff to deal with this sort of problem.

However, medical staff at the hospital will make sure that your father is not discharged until they feel he will be able to manage at home with the assistance available. If necessary, it may be possible to transfer him to a rehabilitation unit for a week or so before he goes home so that he can have additional physiotherapy and occupational therapy to give him the confidence to cope alone.

6. *I have just received a date for my knee replacement operation and find it is about three weeks before a holiday I had already booked. Will I be fit enough to go ahead with my holiday plans?*

It is unlikely that you will be sufficiently mobile to enjoy a holiday so soon after your operation, particularly if you plan to go alone. You may be in hospital for a couple of weeks or more, depending on the progress you make, and will have to continue using walking sticks for several weeks. However, if you are unable to cancel your holiday without serious financial loss, are already familiar with your holiday accommodation and feel that you will be able to manage, you could explain the situation to your doctor or consultant and ask their advice.

7. *I am 45 and have suffered for several years from a painful and increasingly immobile knee joint. The anti-inflammatory drugs which I have been taking for some time have gradually become less effective. My doctor says I am too young to have knee replacement surgery. Is he right and, if so, why?*

Although replaced knee joints can continue to function successfully for up to 15 years or even longer, they do have a finite lifespan. Revision surgery would probably be possible when the replaced joint failed, but because of your relatively young age you are likely to need more than one revision during your lifetime. Each operation causes more damage to the bones and soft tissues and the results are progressively less successful.

On the other hand, if non-surgical treatment, including drugs and physiotherapy, has become ineffective and your quality of life is severely affected, most consultants would be prepared to discuss the possibility of surgery with you. It may therefore be worth asking your doctor to refer you to an orthopaedic consultant for his or her opinion.

8.   I am becoming increasingly disabled because of arthritis in my knees. My consultant has agreed to replace both joints but has said that they cannot be done at the same time. Why do I have to have two separate operations?

Bilateral knee replacement is not undertaken frequently, although there are circumstances under which it would be considered, for example for someone whose knees were both equally severely affected, causing them to be virtually immobile.

Following the replacement of one knee joint, you will need the support of your unoperated leg to help you regain mobility. It would be much more difficult for you to walk and to do the necessary post-operative exercises if both your knee joints were replaced at the same time.

If you have any other co-existent medical condition, such as a weak heart, that is also likely to be considered a contraindication to bilateral total knee replacement. Your consultant will have considered the options and have made the most appropriate decision in your particular circumstances.

9. I had a knee joint replaced about ten years ago but it has recently become painful and I have been told that I need to have revision surgery. What does this entail and is it likely to be as successful as the first operation?

Revision surgery involves the removal and replacement of the primary prostheses. In may be done in one or two stages. A two-stage procedure may be necessary if there is infection in the knee which needs to be cleared up to avoid re-infecting the replaced knee joint. The prostheses would then be removed at one operation and new ones inserted a few weeks later. It may be possible to walk with the aid of walking sticks in the period between the two operations.

If tests prove you to be free of infection, the entire procedure can probably be carried out during a single operation.

Once the original prostheses have been removed, the surgical procedures are similar to those of primary joint replacement. In addition, it may be necessary for the tibia and/or femur to be repaired or reconstructed with bone graft if bone has been lost from them.

It is unlikely that you will regain quite as much movement in your knee after revision, and it is very important that you pay particular attention to doing the post-operative exercises and physiotherapy.

10. My husband is due to have a knee hemi-arthroplasty. What does this operation entail?

Hemi-arthroplasty is similar to total knee replacement except that only one half of a joint is replaced with artificial components. The operation is most likely to involve replacing the ends of the inner side of the tibia and femur. Hemi-arthroplasty is relatively simple to revise to a total knee replacement should this be necessary at a later date.

11. *My mother-in-law has arthritis in most of her joints, but one knee is particularly bad. She recently saw a consultant who said that knee replacement surgery would not be appropriate in her case. Can she ask for a second opinion as I feel that an operation would help her to get around better and to be more independent?*

You can, of course, ask your mother-in-law's doctor to arrange an appointment with another consultant, although his or her opinion may well be the same.

If your mother-in-law's mobility and activity are restricted because of arthritis in other joints, replacing her knee may not lead to any significant improvement in her situation. Surgery may be considered if the knee is very painful and if drug treatment and physiotherapy have become ineffective, but the consultant should have taken these factors into account.

With your mother-in-law's consent, you could write to or ring the consultant she has already seen and ask about the specific reasons why it is felt that knee replacement surgery is inappropriate. It *is* major surgery and the consultant may feel that the possible benefits do not outweigh the risks in her particular case.

12. *I am 78 and have always been quite healthy and active. However, in the last two or three years my arthritic knee has become increasingly painful and disabling. Am I too old for knee replacement surgery?*

Many people in their seventies and even eighties undergo knee replacement surgery. So – all other things being equal – you are certainly not too old to consider this operation. Care will be taken to assess your general state of health and to detect any medical condition you may have which could complicate surgery or the use of anaesthesia or for which particular precautions will have to be taken during or after your operation.

It is certainly worth discussing the possibility of surgery with your doctor as you should not be precluded on the grounds of age alone.

13. My father has recently had a knee joint replaced and was told to do some exercises to regain the movement in it. He is quite forgetful and hates doing the exercises. Will his knee heal and become mobile again even if he doesn't do them?

Your father's knee will probably regain a certain amount of movement, although unless he does the exercises regularly it may always remain flexed to some degree. It is really up to your father whether or not he gains the maximum possible benefit from his operation, and that means regular exercising for at least three months.

If his main reason for having the operation was to deal with pain, and he leads a fairly sedentary life, he may not be as interested in regaining a good range of movement and extension of his knee as someone who wishes to be active. Some people manage quite well with a knee joint which never straightens completely. However, do try to encourage your father to do at least some exercises as his life will certainly be restricted by a permanently flexed knee joint.

14. I have been sent a date for an appointment at a pre-operative assessment clinic. What is it and what will be done at it?

Many hospitals now hold pre-operative assessment clinics a week or two before people are admitted for surgery so that various tests and examinations can be done and their results obtained in good time. The tests should detect any existing infection or a medical condition which could complicate surgery or the use of anaesthesia.

At the clinic, your operation will be explained to you and you will have an opportunity to ask any questions about anything which is not clear to you. You will be given a physical examination and will be asked for details of your medical history and about any other factors which could be relevant, such as any drugs you are taking.

A sample of your blood will be taken to measure its level of haemoglobin and for cross-matching so that blood of the appropriate group can be made ready in case you need a blood transfusion during or after your operation. If the level of haemoglobin is found to be low, indicating anaemia, you will probably be given a course of iron tablets before your operation.

Your urine will be tested to detect the presence of any infection, and you will probably have a chest X-ray and electrocardiogram to make sure that your lungs and heart are functioning properly.

Your knee will also be X-rayed, and you may have one or more scans – a computed tomography and/or magnetic resonance imaging scan.

All these tests provide medical staff with a range of useful information and allow them to build up a clear picture of your general state of health and readiness for surgery.

Case histories

The case histories which follow are not intended to make any specific point. They have been chosen at random as examples of the experiences of different men and women who have undergone total knee replacement.

Although by chance, most of these case histories involve bilateral knee replacement, unilateral operations are much more common.

CASE 1

Emily is 76. Her working life was spent in domestic service, and involved a good deal of kneeling to clean floors. She has had spinal curvature for many years. Following a couple of bad falls onto her knees, her right knee became very painful and she eventually developed deformity of the leg. X-rays showed that the bones at the knee joint were starting to crumble, and it was decided that the knee should be replaced.

Unfortunately, Emily developed a viral infection when the time for her operation arrived, and surgery had to be postponed for a month. However, the operation went well and now, ten years later, apart from some loss of sensation in her lower leg when she walks and stands for long periods, she has no further problems and only returns to hospital for check-ups every couple of years. She uses a walking stick when she goes out and, because the replaced knee has some feeling of instability, she wears a Tubigrip bandage around it during the daytime.

CASE 2

Peter is 45 and has the hereditary disease haemophilia B, which means his blood is unable to clot naturally. It also causes regular episodes of bleeding into the joints — in Peter's case, particularly the knee joints — leading to pain, swelling and inflammation. For many years, Peter had to give himself injections of a clotting agent called Factor 9 to treat these episodes of bleeding when they occurred.

About seven years ago, both his knees had become fixed in a flexed position and he could only walk short distances with the aid of two walking sticks. He became trapped in a vicious circle: as his knees got worse, they bled more; and as they bled more, they got worse. His quality of life was poor and he suffered constant pain.

Peter had been told that he was too young for total knee replacement to be considered and, although surgery might improve his situation, it would be too expensive to provide the daily doses of Factor 9 he would need in the days immediately after each operation to help his blood to clot. However, one day he saw a different surgeon at the hospital who thought that knee replacement would be feasible and suggested that both knees be replaced at the same time, thus halving the cost of providing Factor 9 after two separate operations.

Peter experienced quite severe pain for two or three days after the operation, during which time he used a patient-controlled analgesia machine. He was helped to get out of bed and to take a few steps on the second day after his operation, and remained in hospital for three and a half weeks, doing daily physiotherapy.

Some 18 months later, he has had no further episodes of bleeding into his knees, although he continues to have to inject Factor 9 when other joints bleed. He still has hydrotherapy every couple of weeks and does at least half an hour's exercising at home each day. He can now straighten one of his knees completely, and the other is only slightly stiff. He can walk without the support of walking sticks for the first time in many years, and has no further pain in his knees. His life has been transformed by his operation and he is grateful to have had the chance to enjoy it while still young.

CASE 3

Gloria is 57. She has suffered from rheumatoid arthritis for some 14 years. After numerous falls some years ago, her right hip became very painful, she began to have difficulty walking, and she underwent total hip replacement five years ago. Soon after her right hip was replaced, her left hip became painful and made loud cracking noises, and it too was eventually replaced.

Some time later, Gloria's knees began to swell and fluid had to be withdrawn from them at regular intervals. Eventually, both knees became permanently flexed and very painful. She was admitted to hospital for a week for daily withdrawal of fluid and for bed rest, but the problems returned shortly afterwards. An X-ray showed that the bones of both knees were significantly worn. Gloria spent a year in a wheelchair, housebound and in considerable pain, and she was admitted for surgery to replace both her knees about six months ago.

She was in hospital for ten days, and could bend and straighten both her knees by the time she was discharged. She is now quite mobile although she cannot walk very far without becoming out of breath. She uses a walking stick when she goes out, as much for the feeling of security it provides as for support. She has no more pain from her knees (or hips) and is very happy with the results of her operations.

CASE 4

Edith is 86. She has suffered with arthritis for several years, which particularly affected her knees. By the time she underwent bilateral knee replacement about three years ago, her knees were swollen and inflamed, she was housebound, unable to walk, and in considerable pain.

After her operation, Edith spent several weeks in hospital and was then transferred to an elderly persons' home as it was felt that she was no longer able to manage alone. She seemed to be making good progress, but about a month after she had settled in to her new home, her carer noticed that her right knee was very red and swollen. The doctor gave Edith a course of antibiotics, but when pus started to leak from the scar, she was returned to hospital for further treatment for an infection and for revision surgery to her right knee. However, once in hospital, it was decided that revision surgery would not be possible, so the primary prosthesis was removed and a metal pin was inserted to fuse the bones of the knee together.

When Edith left hospital, some two months later, she was fairly mobile and able to walk with a walking frame. She had a plaster cast around her knee, but it had to be removed when her foot became very swollen and she developed an ulcer where it rubbed on her ankle. She then wore a knee brace for several months.

She cannot bend her right knee at all, and the muscles in her leg have tended to waste through lack of use, while those in her left leg have become quite strong. Because Edith now stands with her weight on her left foot, she has experienced some problems, including an ulcer on the underside of a toe, which took some time to heal. However, she no longer suffers any pain from her knees and is able to do most things for herself, including dressing and pottering around her room and, with the aid of her walking frame, around the home in which she lives. She can also manage to go up and down a few stairs when necessary.

Medical terms

Abrasion   A damaged area of skin where the surface has been scraped or worn away by rubbing.

Abscess   A collection of pus secondary to localised infection. Pus is a fluid containing dead cells, fragments of tissue and sometimes bacteria, which forms as a result of inflammation.

Adhesion   A piece of tissue uniting parts which are normally separate. Adhesions may form as the result of inflammation and can restrict movement, for example if they form between two bones at a joint.

Allergy   An abnormal reaction to a substance. An allergic reaction can be mild, causing an itchy rash, or severe, leading to fainting, vomiting, loss of consciousness or death.

Allograft   A graft between two individuals of the same species.

Alloy   A mixture of two or more metals.

Anaemia   A condition caused by deficiency of red cells or haemoglobin in the blood.

Anaesthesia   The absence of sensation.

Anaesthetic   A drug which causes loss of sensation in part or all of the body.

Anaesthetist   A doctor who is trained in the administration of anaesthetics.

Analgesic   A drug which blocks the sensation of pain; a painkiller.

Ankylosing spondylitis   An inflammatory disease of the spine which causes soft tissue calcification and immobility of the affected parts of the vertebral column (bamboo spine). It may also affect the hips and other large joints.

Antagonistic muscles   Pairs of muscles which control the movement of limbs by acting in opposition to one another: contraction of one muscle of the pair produces movement in one direction, while contraction of the other produces movement in the opposite direction.

Antibiotic   A substance which kills bacteria or prevents them replicating.

Anticoagulant   A substance which thins the blood and prevents it from clotting.

Anti-embolism stockings   Stockings sometimes worn during an operation and during any period of immobilisation post-operatively. The stockings assist the circulation of blood in the legs and reputedly help to prevent blood clots forming.

Anti-emetic   A drug which helps to reduce feelings of sickness.

Arthritis   Inflammation of a joint.

Arthrodesis   Surgical fusion of bones to produce a completely rigid, inflexible joint.

Arthropathy   Any disease affecting a joint.

Arthroplasty   Surgical reconstruction of a joint, with or without an implant.

Articular cartilage   Cartilage which covers the articulating surfaces of a synovial joint, such as the knee joint.

Aseptic loosening   Loosening of an artificial component in a replaced joint which is due to something other than infection.

Aspiration   The withdrawal of fluid or gas from a body cavity using suction.

Atrophy   Wasting away due to lack of nourishment or use.

Autograft   A graft of skin or of other tissue taken from one part of the body to correct a defect in another part of the same individual.

Autologous blood transfusion   The re-infusion of blood which is collected from part of the body, filtered to remove any debris, and re-introduced via a cannula, usually in the arm.

Biceps femoris muscle   One of the hamstring muscles of the thigh which controls flexion. It has two points of attachment, at the pelvis and at the head of the fibula.

Bilateral knee replacement An operation to replace both knee joints.

Biocompatible Indicates that the material or substance is biologically acceptable to the human body.

Biological fixation A technique whereby a prosthesis is coated with a porous layer, such as cobalt chrome beads or titanium mesh, to induce the growth of bone into it.

Biomechanics The science of forces acting on an organism or on part of an organism.

Biopsy The surgical removal of a piece of tissue from a living body for examination under a microscope to assist or confirm a diagnosis.

Blood transfusion The transfer of blood from one individual (the donor) to another (the recipient) which is sometimes necessary after surgery when substantial volumes of blood have been lost. Blood from the recipient is cross-matched pre-operatively to make sure that blood of the same type is transfused. The transfusion of incompatible blood can lead to serious complications.

Bone bank A place where bone is stored in very cold freezers for use in grafting.

Bone stock The quality and quantity of bone.

Cannula A very fine tube or needle which is now usually made of plastic. (Metal or glass was used in the past.) Fluids can be introduced into or removed from the body through an intravenous cannula inserted into a vein, usually in the back of the hand. Intravenous cannulas are also used to administer anaesthetic drugs during an operation.

Cardiovascular Relating to the heart and blood vessels.

Cartilage A specialised body tissue which is firm but flexible and which, for example, covers the articulating surfaces of bone in a synovial joint.

Catheter   A thin tube used to withdraw fluid from or introduce it into the body.

Cauterise   To burn a part with heat or some other agent. During surgery, bleeding from the severed ends of small blood vessels is stopped by sealing them with the tip an instrument heated by an electric current.

Cement-fixed prosthesis   An artificial implant which is fixed in place using cement.

Cementless prosthesis   An artificial implant which is fixed in place without the use of cement, for example one designed for biological fixation.

Centrifugation   A process whereby a liquid is rotated at very high speed to separate it from another liquid or from a solid.

Ceramic   A substance produced by heating clay and minerals to a high temperature to give it strength and make it hard. It may be used as an articular surface or as a bioactive coating in joint implants, although it is not commonly employed in knee replacement.

Cobalt chrome   A tough, malleable alloy of the hard metals cobalt and chrome.

Complication   A condition which occurs as the result of another disease or condition. It may also be an unwanted side-effect of treatment.

Component   An artificial part used to replace a body part; a prosthesis or implant.

Computed tomography (CT)   A scan which takes X-rays through 'slices' of the body. The images are interpreted by a computer to build up a three-dimensional picture.

Condyle   A rounded articular surface at the end of a bone.

Congenital   Present from birth.

Connective tissue   Fibrous tissue which connects and supports organs within the body.

Consent form   A form which patients must sign before surgery to confirm that they understand what is involved in their operation and give their consent for it to take place. Signing the form also gives consent for the use of anaesthetic drugs and any other procedures which doctors feel to be necessary.

Constraint　The degree of freedom of movement, for example of a prosthesis.

Consultant　A fully trained doctor with at least 10 to 15 years' experience who specialises in a particular type of medicine. A hospital consultant will head a team (or 'firm') of doctors in a particular field of medicine.

Continuous passive motion machine　A frame-like structure of adjustable length which moves continuously up and down. It may be used after knee surgery to move the leg passively and to aid wound healing. It cannot, however, replace the need for active movement of the limb.

Contracture　Deformity caused by shortening of muscle and soft tissues around the joint.

Cross-match　Matching of donor and recipient blood to ensure that blood of the same group is given on transfusion.

Cryotherapy　The application of ice to reduce swelling, inflammation or bruising.

Day-case surgery　Surgery for which a patient is in hospital for one day only, with no overnight stay.

Debridement　The process of 'cleaning out' fragments of cartilage and other debris which may accompany knee joint surgery.

Deep vein thrombosis (DVT)　A blood clot in a deep vein, often in the lower leg or pelvis.

Degenerative disease　Any disease involving the breaking down of an organ or tissue, thereby affecting its form and/or function.

Diagnosis　The identification of a disease based on its symptoms and signs.

Diathermy　A method of generating heat by means of a high-frequency electric current. It is used in surgery to destroy diseased tissue or to stop bleeding from damaged blood vessels.

Direct closure   The drawing together of the edges of a wound with stitches.

Discharge letter   A letter given to patients leaving hospital (or sent directly from the hospital) to deliver to their family doctor. It gives details of the treatment they have received and any follow-up required.

Dislocation   Complete displacement of one bone in relation to another at a joint, or of one component of a prosthesis in relation to the other.

Dissection   The separation or division of structures by cutting or tearing the connective tissue between them which is done during surgical procedures or for anatomical study.

Distension   The act of enlarging or dilating.

Diuretic   Any substance which increases the volume of urine produced.

Drain   A tube which is inserted near a wound to drain excess blood and fluid into a bag or bottle.

Drip/Intravenous infusion   A tube through which specially balanced saline or sugar solution is administered into a vein in the arm to replace fluid lost from the body after an operation or injury.

Dura (mater)   The tough outer membrane which surrounds the brain and spinal cord in a protective sheath.

Electrocardiogram (ECG)   The activity of the heart recorded as a series of electrical wave patterns.

Electrocautery   The application of the electrically heated tip of an instrument to the ends of blood vessels in order to stop them bleeding.

Embolus (plural: **emboli**)   A piece of a blood clot (or air bubble) which has broken away and can pass through the blood vessels. If it lodges in a vital organ, such as the lung, it can have fatal consequences.

Epidural anaesthetic   An anaesthetic drug which is injected outside the dura into the space around the nerves in the back. It causes numbness in the legs and groin which lasts for three to five hours. Epidurals are used for pain relief and/or to produce loss of sensation during surgery to the legs or lower body.

Erythema   Redness due to increased blood flow.

Excision   Removal by cutting.

Excision arthroplasty   The surgical removal of a joint.

Extension   Straightening, for example of a bent limb.

External rotation   Rotation away from the body, for example of a limb.

Femoral component   An artificial implant inserted to replace part of the thigh bone.

Femur   The thigh bone.

Fibrosis   The development of excessive fibrous tissue.

Fibula   The narrow, outer bone of the lower leg which extends from just below the knee to the ankle. The fibula does not form part of the knee joint.

Fixed Price Care   The system used by some private hospitals whereby a fixed price is quoted for a particular type of operation and some of the hospitalisation costs associated with it.

Flexion   The bending of a joint so that the two parts connected by it come together.

Flexion contracture   Shortening of muscles and soft tissues which produces fixed flexion of a joint, i.e. an inability to extend it fully.

Flowtron   A large, inflatable splint which was originally developed to treat oedema but which can also be placed around a limb to stretch it. Flowtrons are sometimes used following knee replacement surgery to aid extension of the knee joint.

Foot pump   A pump which is usually placed at the end of the bed and attached to special boots made of a soft, foam-like material. A pocket under each foot automatically inflates and deflates to assist the circulation of blood in the legs during periods of immobility. Although in some hospitals foot pumps are now used routinely following some types of surgery, their role in helping to reduce the post-operative risk of thrombosis is still being evaluated.

Foreign body reaction   The body's reaction to the presence of some substance which is not usually found within it. Large inflammatory cells accumulate around the foreign material in an attempt to seal it off and isolate it.

Fracture   A break, particularly of a bone.

Gait   Way of walking.

Gastrointestinal tract   The stomach and intestines.

General anaesthetic   A drug which induces loss of consciousness and abolishes the sensation of pain in all parts of the body.

Graft   A piece of tissue removed from one site and placed at another to repair a defect resulting from an operation, accident or disease. The tissue can be taken from the same or another individual.

Haematoma   A blood-filled swelling. A haematoma can form in a wound after an operation if blood continues to leak from a blood vessel. If the blood spreads in the tissues, it appears as a bruise.

Haemoglobin   An iron-containing pigment in red blood cells which carries oxygen molecules around the body. As a good supply of oxygen is vital for wound healing, it is important that there is an adequate level of haemoglobin in the blood after surgery.

Haemophilia   An inherited disease, transmitted by women but normally affecting only men, in which the mechanism of blood clotting is faulty, leading to uncontrolled bleeding when a blood vessel is severed.

Haemorrhage   Bleeding.

Hamstring muscles   A group of muscles in the lower limb comprising the biceps femoris, semitendinosus and semimembranosus muscles.

Hemi-arthroplasty   The replacement of one half of each of the bones of a joint with artificial implants.

Heparin   A substance which occurs naturally in the body and which helps to prevent the blood clotting. It may be given by injection before and after surgery to people who are at particular risk of developing blood clots.

Heterotopic bone formation   The development of bone at a site at which it would not normally occur.

High-density polyethylene   A very strong plastic with good wear properties which is used to make some types of prostheses for joint replacement.

Hinge joint   A synovial joint between two bones which only moves in one plane, for example the elbow joint.

Histological examination   The microscopic examination of a sample of tissue which has been taken from the body by biopsy.

Hydrotherapy   Treatment involving the use of water.

Hydroxyapatite   A chemical compound, containing calcium phosphate, from which bone salts are derived.

Hypothermia   A condition in which the temperature of the body is abnormally low.

Ibuprofen   A type of non-steroidal anti-inflammatory drug.

Incision   A cut or wound made by a sharp instrument, such as during an operation.

Incontinence   Lack of voluntary control over the discharge of urine or faeces.

Indomethacin   A non-steroidal anti-inflammatory drug with pain-killing properties.

Induction agent   A drug used in anaesthesia to bring on loss of consciousness.

Inhalational anaesthetic   An anaesthetic given as a mixture of gases which is inhaled, usually to maintain anaesthesia.

Inflammation   The response of a tissue to injury or infection which involves the rush of blood and white blood cells to the affected part, causing redness, swelling and pain.

Internal rotation   Rotation towards the central axis of the body, for example of a limb.

Interpositional arthroplasty An operation to interpose a material between the ends of bones or the surfaces of a joint to keep them apart.

Intravenous anaesthetic A general anaesthetic drug which is injected via a cannula into a vein, usually in the back of the hand.

Intra-operative Occurring during an operation.

Joint The junction of two or more bones which enables them to move relative to each other.

Joint cavity The space between the bones of a joint which is filled with synovial fluid; synovial cavity.

Ligament A tough, flexible strand of fibrous tissue which connects bones and contributes towards the stability of a joint.

Local anaesthetic An anaesthetic which numbs the area of the body around which it is injected.

Local injection An injection of a substance which remains confined to one area and is not distributed throughout the body.

Locomotor system All the parts of the body involved in movement.

Lymph A pale-coloured fluid which flows within the lymphatic vessels of the body and is eventually returned to the blood. It contains disease-fighting cells called lymphocytes.

Lymphocyte A type of white blood cell involved in fighting disease in the body.

Lymphoedema A condition in which the lymphatic drainage of part of the body is impaired, causing swelling, tightness of the skin and pain as the lymph collects.

Magnetic resonance imaging (MRI) The use of a large magnet to produce a magnetic field in individual cells of the body. An energy field is applied which affects the alignment of atoms within the cells and causes them to emit a signal which is detected by a computer and interpreted as an image of the body. The procedure is very useful for visualising soft tissues which are not seen on routine X-rays.

Maintenance agent   A drug used during an operation to maintain the state of general anaesthesia.

Manipulation   The manual movement of a joint beyond the extent to which it can be actively moved.

Metastatic infection   Infection which has spread from a primary site to another part of the body, either directly or via the blood or lymphatic vessels.

Monomer   A compound of low molecular weight which can be linked with units of the same compound to form a substance with different properties – a polymer.

Morphine   A drug derived from opium which has several effects on the body, including that of providing good pain relief. It may also cause vomiting and is therefore usually given in conjunction with an anti-emetic. Its effects on the nervous system include damping down the movements of the intestine, which may lead to constipation.

Nasogastric tube   A tube inserted via a nostril after some operations to drain the stomach contents and prevent vomiting. A smaller version is sometimes used to introduce a specially balanced fluid into the stomach to feed patients who are unable to eat.

National Health Service (NHS)   The system of medical care, set up in Britain in 1948, under which medical treatment is mostly funded by taxation.

Nausea   A feeling of sickness.

Necrosis   The death of tissue.

Nerve palsy   Loss of function in some part of the body due to damage to its nerves.

Neuroma   A swelling of nerve cells and nerve fibres.

Neuropathy   A condition involving the destruction or degeneration of the tissue of the central or peripheral nerves, caused by drugs or metabolic or vascular disturbance.

Nil by mouth   A term used to mean that no food or drink should be swallowed in the hours before an operation.

Nodule   A small swelling of cells.

Non-steroidal anti-inflammatory drug (NSAID)   A drug which suppresses inflammation but which is not a steroid, for example indomethacin and ibuprofen.

Obesity   An excessive amount of fat in the body. This term is non-specific and is being replaced by a figure calculated from height and weight measurements, known as the **body mass index**.

Occupational therapist   Someone trained to assist people in their recovery from disease, injury or surgery by means of mental or physical activity.

Oedema   Swelling caused by an excessive amount of fluid in the spaces between the cells of tissues. It may occur as a result of inflammation, an allergic reaction or obstruction of the lymphatic or blood vessels.

Oestrogen   A hormone which is produced in the ovaries and the adrenal glands above the kidneys and which stimulates sexual development in women as well as changes in the lining of the womb during the menstrual cycle.

One-stage revision   The removal of the components of a replaced knee and the insertion of new ones during a single operation.

Orthopaedic consultant   A surgeon who specialises in disease and deformities of the parts of the body involved in locomotion, for example the muscles and bones.

Orthopaedic surgery   Surgery to correct abnormalities, diseases or injury of the parts of the body involved in movement.

Osseo-integration   The process of growth of bone into another substance.

Ossification   The formation of bone.

Osteoarthritis   Disorder of a joint which causes it to degenerate. It is often age related but may result from severe or repeated injury or from abnormal alignment. Osteoarthritis of the knee may be a result of obesity.

Osteolysis   The breaking down and absorption of bone or the loss of calcium from it.

Osteophyte   Outgrowth of bone at the edge of a joint.

Osteoporosis   An increase in the porosity of bone due to loss of minerals from it. It may occur with increasing age, particularly in post-menopausal women, and makes the bones brittle and prone to fracture.

Osteotome   A chisel-like surgical instrument used to cut bone.

Osteotomy   An operation which involves cutting through bone. It may be done to realign bones and to redistribute the load through the adjacent joint.

Patella   The bone which lies in front of the knee joint; the knee cap.

Patella dislocation   Displacement of the knee cap, usually to the side (laterally).

Patient-controlled analgesia (PCA)   The administration of pain-killing drugs via a cannula, inserted into a vein in the hand or arm, which is controlled by the patient. A preset dosage of the drug is delivered by a pump whenever the patient presses a button on the PCA machine.

Physiotherapy   The use of physical measures to build muscle strength, correct deformity and restore function after disease, injury or surgery.

Polyethylene   A tough, flexible, synthetic resin often used to make joint prostheses.

Polymer   A compound comprising repeated units of one or more simpler compounds.

Polymethylmethacrylate   A chemical constituent of bone cement used to fix joint prostheses into the existing bone.

Post-menopausal   Following the menopause.

Post-operative   Following an operation.

Pre-medication ('pre-med.')   A drug which is given before another drug, for example one given an hour or two before an operation to relax the patient before anaesthesia is started.

Pre-operative   Before an operation.

Pre-operative assessment/Pre-clerking admission procedure
A procedure used in some hospitals whereby patients attend an appointment a few days or weeks before an operation for any necessary pre-operative tests, such as blood tests and ECGs, the results of which are thus available by the time they are admitted for surgery.

Press-fit prosthesis   An uncemented artificial joint component which can be pressed into place.

Pressure sore   A sore which can develop as a result of continuous pressure being exerted on part of the body, for example during long periods of lying in bed. Pressure sores tend to occur on parts of the body where weight-bearing is greatest, for example the heels, buttocks, elbows etc. when lying on the back, or anywhere which comes in contact with the bedsheet when lying on the side. Predisposing factors are moisture, friction and pressure, but sores may still develop despite precautions being taken to keep the skin clean and dry and to change position regularly. In severe cases pressure sores can ulcerate, sometimes with serious consequences.

Primary knee replacement   An operation to replace the bones of the knee joint for the first time.

Prognosis   An opinion about the probable course and final outcome of a disease which is made when all the known facts are considered.

Prophylactic   Something used to prevent a disease or condition developing.

Prosthesis   An artificial part.

Pulmonary embolism   A blood clot or air bubble which blocks the blood vessels in the lung.

Pyrexia   A fever.

Quadriceps femoris muscle   The muscle at the front of the thigh which is inserted into the patella and which controls extension of the knee joint.

Reamer   A small surgical instrument used to make or enlarge a cavity in bone, for example to insert a prosthesis during a knee replacement operation.

Recovery room   A ward near the operating theatre to which patients are taken after surgery so that they can be closely watched while they recover from a general anaesthetic.

Reduction   Restoration of tissue to its natural position.

Referred pain   Pain felt in one part of the body which arises as a result of damage or disease in another part.

Regional anaesthesia   Anaesthesia of a specific area of the body.

Rehabilitation   Training to restore the use of a part of the body which has been lost or reduced following injury, disease or surgery.

Rehabilitation unit   A special unit in some hospitals where people can stay for a short period following an operation such as knee replacement if they have not regained sufficient confidence and mobility to manage at home by the time they are discharged. Daily sessions with a physiotherapist and occupational therapist are amongst the procedures used to encourage the resumption of normal daily activities.

Resection   The surgical removal of tissue or an organ.

Revision surgery   Surgery which is repeated due to the failure of an earlier operation.

Rheumatoid arthritis   Inflammation, typically of multiple joints, causing pain, weakness and eventually deformity and loss of function. Its causes are unknown.

Secondary osteoarthritis   Damage to the joints which continues even though the primary disease has burned itself out.

Semimembranosus muscle   One of the hamstring muscles which runs between the pelvis and the protruberance at the top of the tibia.

Semitendinosus muscle   One of the hamstring muscles which runs between the pelvis and the upper part of the tibia.

Sepsis   Infection caused by pus-producing bacteria.

Septicaemia   Severe infection caused by large numbers of bacteria in the blood which multiply and spread; blood poisoning.

Seroma   A collection of clear fluid, such as lymph, which may develop following an operation. If persistent, the fluid can be drawn off with a needle.

Shaft   The long, cylindrical part of a bone.

Side-effect   An effect other than that desired which results from the use of a drug or other form of treatment.

Sign   Something a doctor looks for as an indication of disease, such as redness or swelling.

Skin graft   A piece of skin taken from one site on the body to replace that which has been lost because of injury or surgery at another site.

Spinal anaesthetic   An anaesthetic which is injected between the vertebrae of the spine into the space around the nerves in the back. It causes numbness in the legs and groin which lasts for three to five hours.

Stasis   The slowing down or cessation of flow of a fluid. Blood stasis causes pooling of blood within a blood vessel.

Steroid   One of a group of naturally occurring substances in the body which includes some hormones.

Subluxation   Incomplete dislocation of a joint.

Surgical manipulation   Movement of a joint to break down adhesions which are preventing it moving normally. The procedure is performed by a surgeon while the patient is anaesthetised. It needs to be done within about four to six weeks after the operation, before the development of scar tissue makes it more difficult and more prone to causing damage.

Suture   A surgical stitch or row of stitches.

Symptom   Something experienced by a patient which indicates a disturbance of normal body function, for example pain or nausea.

Synovial fluid The fluid secreted by the synovial membrane of a joint which is present in the space between its bones and which nourishes and lubricates their ends.

Synovial joint A mobile joint, the bones of which are separated by synovial fluid.

Synovitis Inflammation of the synovial membrane of a joint. It is usually accompanied by the collection of synovial fluid within the joint cavity, and thus by swelling.

Synovium The membrane around a joint cavity which secretes synovial fluid.

Thrombo-embolic deterrent stockings (TEDS) *See* Anti-embolism stockings.

Thromboplastin A substance which is released into the bloodstream when blood is shed and which plays a role in the formation of a blood clot.

Thrombosis The coagulation of blood within a vein or artery which produces a blood clot.

Thrombus A blood clot which remains within the blood vessel in which it forms.

Tibia The long bone on the inside of the lower leg which articulates at the knee joint with the lower surface of the femur. Below the knee, it also articulates with the other calf bone – the fibula.

Tibial component An artificial prosthesis inserted to replace part of the tibia.

Titanium A metal present in certain ores.

Titanium alloy A combination of the metal titanium with iron or copper.

Total knee joint replacement The surgical removal of parts of the femur and tibia and their replacement with artificial components.

Tourniquet An instrument used to compress a limb and interrupt its blood supply, thus preventing haemorrhage from a wound or loss of blood during an operation.

Toxicity   The quality of being poisonous.

Tracheal tube   A tube which is inserted into the windpipe (the trachea) to keep the airways to the lungs open during the process of anaesthesia.

Trauma   Injury.

Trial component   A component used during a knee replacement operation to assess the optimal size of prosthesis that fits the resected bone ends and provides stability.

Two-stage revision   Revision surgery done in two separate operations, sometimes to allow for treatment of infection before new prostheses are inserted. The primary components are removed at the first operation; the bone is reconstructed and new components are inserted during the second – often six weeks or more later.

Ulcer   A lesion of the skin in which the surface layers have been destroyed, exposing the deeper tissues.

Urinalysis   The analysis of urine to detect the presence of certain chemicals and/or of bacteria.

Urinary catheter   A narrow tube inserted through the urethra into the bladder to drain urine from it. It may be used for a short period after surgery until urine can be passed spontaneously again.

Urinary retention   Retention of urine in the bladder caused by obstruction to its flow or weakness of the muscles of the bladder wall.

Valve   A device which regulates the flow of liquid. The valves present in the veins ensure that blood flows in one direction only (towards the heart). They are composed of small projections of tissue called **valve cusps.**

Warfarin   An anticoagulant which may be used to treat thrombosis by thinning the blood and helping to dissolve the blood clot.

Wear debris   Small particles which are rubbed off the articulating surfaces of prostheses as a result of the friction between them. The particles can set up an inflammatory reaction, causing breakdown and absorption of the surrounding bone, and eventually loosening of the prostheses themselves.

Xenograft   A graft between a donor and a recipient of different species.

X-ray   A type of electromagnetic radiation of short wavelength which is able to pass through opaque structures. It can be used in diagnosis, by allowing the visualisation of internal structures and organs of the body, or in higher doses as therapy to destroy malignant cells.

Useful addresses

There are various organisations in most countries throughout the world which provide advice, information and, in some cases, practical support. A few of those in the UK are listed here, but the addresses of arthritis societies or foundations can be found in your telephone directory. Your hospital or health department should also be able to supply details of any other useful organisations in your area.

Disabled Living Centres/Independent Living Centres

There are centres throughout the UK, the addresses of which can be obtained from a telephone directory or from the Disabled Living Foundation (see below). They provide free and independent advice about the assistance available, both practical and financial, and at many you can see and try out various aids before deciding whether to buy. Many of the staff are physiotherapists or occupational therapists.

The Disabled Living Foundation

380–384 Harrow Road
London W9 2HU
Telephone: 0171 289 6111

The Disabled Living Foundation provides advice on aids and appliances for the home.

Mobility Advice and Vehicle Information Service
Department of Transport
TRL
Crowthorne
Berkshire RG45 6AU
Telephone: 01344 770456

This service was set up by the Department of Transport and provides assessment of driving ability and practical advice on possible car adaptations for both drivers and passengers with disability. Contact the service at Crowthorne for the addresses of other centres around the country.

The Arthritis and Rheumatism Council
Copeman House
St Mary's Court
St Mary's Gate
Chesterfield
Derbyshire S41 7TD
Telephone: 01246 558033

This is a charitable organisation which funds research projects into rheumatic diseases and produces a range of leaflets giving explanations and practical advice.

Arthritis Care
18 Stephenson Way
London NW1 2HD
Telephone: 0171 916 1500 (open 10 a.m. to 4 p.m., Monday to Friday)
Helpline: Freephone 0800 289170 (open 12 a.m. to 4 p.m., Monday to Friday)

Free confidential advice and information are available, by letter or phone, from a counselling team.

The Royal Association for Disability & Rehabilitation
25 Mortimer Street
London W1N 8AB
Telephone: 0171 250 3222

Information and advice can be obtained from this national organisation, including details of national and local groups and of the entitlement to various social services etc. of those with particular disabilities.

Department of Social Services
There may be community occupational therapists based at your local Department of Social Services who can give you advice and home assessment, although there may be some delay before an appointment can be made for you. The address and phone number of your local DSS will be in your telephone directory.

How to complain

If you are unhappy about anything that has occurred – or, indeed, that has not occurred – during your stay in hospital and wish to make a complaint, there are several possible paths to follow. However, before you set the complaints machinery in motion, you should give careful thought to what is involved. Once a formal complaint has been made against a doctor and the complaints procedure has begun, there is little chance of stopping it.

If you think you have a genuine grievance, do try to talk to the person concerned, explaining as clearly and unemotionally as possible what it is that you feel has gone wrong. If you do not feel able to discuss things directly, you can always present your case in a letter.

The vast majority of doctors – family doctors and those who work in hospitals – are dedicated, conscientious and hard working. They really do have their patients' best interests at heart, and many work very long hours each week, night and day. A complaint against a doctor is usually a devastating blow, which can cause considerable stress. Of course, if something has gone wrong during your medical treatment, you may also have suffered stress and unhappiness, but before you make an official complaint, do consider whether your doctor's actions have really warranted what many would see as a 'kick in the teeth'.

The best approach is to make a polite and reasoned enquiry to the person concerned. However angry or irritated you may feel, a complaint made aggressively is unlikely to achieve much.

The following brief sections explain how to make an official complaint in the UK. Leaflets and other information giving details of all the appropriate councils and complaints procedures and how they work can be obtained from your hospital or local health authority. If you have any problems with the offices mentioned below, information about what to do and who to go to for help is available from Citizens' Advice Bureaus and Community Health Councils.

HOSPITAL STAFF

If your complaint concerns something that has happened during your stay in hospital and for some reason you are unable to approach the person directly concerned, you can talk to the ward sister or charge nurse, the hospital doctor on your ward, or the senior manager for the department or ward. If they cannot deal with your complaint directly, they will be able to refer you to the appropriate person.

THE GENERAL MANAGER

If you are intimidated by the thought of speaking to one of the people mentioned above, you can write to the hospital's General Manager, sometimes called the Director of Operations or Chief Executive. The General Manager has responsibility for the way the hospital is run.

The Government's Patients' Charter states that anyone making a complaint about an NHS service must receive a 'full and prompt written reply from the Chief Executive or General Manager'. You should therefore receive an immediate response to your letter, and your complaint should be fully investigated by a senior manager.

The hospital switchboard, or any member of the medical or clerical staff at the hospital, should be able to give you the General Manager's name and office address. If you would prefer to do so, you can make an appointment to speak to him or her, rather than writing a letter.

Depending on how serious your complaint is, you should receive either a full report of the investigation into it or regular letters telling you what is happening until such a report can be made. Do make sure you keep copies of all letters you write and receive concerning your complaint.

DISTRICT HEALTH AUTHORITY

If the treatment you require is not available in your area, or the waiting list is very long, your local District Health Authority may be able to arrange for you to have treatment elsewhere where waiting lists are shorter, if this is what you want. The District Health Authority is able to deal with complaints concerning the provision of services, rather than with those resulting from something going wrong with your treatment.

COMMUNITY HEALTH COUNCIL

Independent advice and assistance can be obtained from your local Community Health Council. Someone from the Community Health Council will be able to explain the complaints procedures to you, help you to write letters to the hospital, and also come with you to any meetings arranged between hospital representatives and yourself. Again, the address of the Community Health Council for your area can be obtained from a hospital or local telephone directory.

REGIONAL MEDICAL OFFICER

If your complaint concerns the standard of *clinical* treatment you received in hospital, and the paths you have already taken have not led to a satisfactory conclusion, you can take it to the Regional Medical Officer for your area.

FAMILY HEALTH SERVICES AUTHORITY

Family doctors are now encouraged to have their own 'in-house' complaints services, but a complaint about your family doctor which you have been unable to sort out by this means can be reported to the Family Health Services Authority. Such complaints should be made within 13 weeks of the incident occurring. Again, your local Community Health Council will be able to give you advice and help you make your complaint and write letters etc.

HEALTH SERVICE COMMISSIONER

If all else has failed, you can take your complaint to the Health Service Commissioner, who is responsible to Parliament and independent of both the NHS and the Government.

The Health Service Commissioner can deal with complaints made by individuals about the failure of an NHS authority to provide the service it should – a failure which has caused actual hardship or injustice. You must have taken your complaint up with your local health authority first, but if you have not received a satisfactory response within a reasonable time, write to the Health Service Commissioner enclosing copies of *all* the relevant letters and documents as well as giving details of the incident itself. The Health Commissioner is not able to investigate complaints about clinical treatment.

You must contact the Health Service Commissioner within *one* year of the incident occurring, unless there is some valid reason why you have been unable to do so.

There is a separate Health Service Commissioner for each country within the United Kingdom.

Health Service Commissioner for England
Church House
Great Smith Street
London SW1P 3BW
Telephone: 0171 276 2035

Health Service Commissioner for Scotland
Second Floor
11 Melville Crescent
Edinburgh EH3 7LU
Telephone: 0131 225 7465

Health Service Commissioner for Wales
4th Floor Pearl Assurance House
Greyfriars Road
Cardiff CF1 3AG
Telephone: 01222 394621

Office of the Northern Ireland Commissioner for Complaints
33 Wellington Place
Belfast BT1 6HN
Telephone: 01232 233821

TAKING LEGAL ACTION

The legal path is likely to be an expensive one, and should be a last resort rather than a starting point.

In theory, everyone has a right to take legal action. However, unless you have very little money and are entitled to Legal Aid, or a great deal of money, you are unlikely to be able to afford this costly process. The outcome of legal action can never be assured, and the possible cost if you lose your case should be borne in mind.

If you do think you have grounds for compensation for injury caused to you as a result of negligence, advice can be sought from:

The Association for the Victims of Medical Accidents (AVMA)
1 London Road
Forest Hill
London SE23 3TP
Telephone: 0181 291 2793.

Someone from the AVMA will be able to give you free and confidential legal advice about whether or not you have a case worth pursuing. They will also be able to recommend solicitors with training in medical law who may be prepared to represent you.

SUMMARY

Do tell nursing or other medical staff if you are not happy about *any* aspect of your care in hospital. They may be able to deal with your complaint immediately. But do remember, if the matter is a serious one, or if you are not satisfied with the response you receive, you are entitled to pursue it through all the levels that exist to deal with such problems.

Index